Michael
Ontimisiens

Variants of Ventricular Preexcitation

RECOGNITION AND TREATMENT

Variants of Ventricular Preexcitation

RECOGNITION AND TREATMENT

Eduardo Back Sternick, MD, PhD

Biocor Instituto
Arrhythmia and Electrophysiology Unit
Belo Horizonte
Minas Gerais, Brazil

Hein JJ Wellens, MD, PhD, FACC, FESC, FAHA, FRCP

University of Maastricht
Professor of Cardiology
Maastricht, Netherlands

Blackwell
Futura

Published by Blackwell Publishing
Blackwell Futura is an imprint of Blackwell Publishing

Blackwell Publishing, Inc., 350 Main Street, Malden, Massachusetts 02148-5020, USA
Blackwell Publishing Ltd, 9600 Garsington Road, Oxford OX4 2DQ, UK
Blackwell Science Asia Pty Ltd, 550 Swanston Street, Carlton, Victoria 3053, Australia

First published 2006

1 2006

ISBN-13: 978-1-4051-48436
ISBN-10: 1-4051-48438

Library of Congress Cataloging-in-Publication Data

Sternick, Eduardo Back.
Variants of ventricular preexcitation : recognition and treatment / Eduardo Back Sternick, Hein J. Wellens.
p. ; cm.
Includes bibliographical references and index.
ISBN-13: 978-1-4051-4843-6 (alk. paper)
ISBN-10: 1-4051-4843-8 (alk. paper)
1. Wolff-Parkinson-White syndrome. 2. Excitation (Physiology)
[DNLM: 1. Pre-Excitation, Mahaim-Type. 2. Myocardium–pathology. WG 330 S839v 2006]
I. Wellens, H. J. J. II. Title.
RC685.W6S74 2006
616.1′24–dc22

2006007279

A catalogue record for this title is available from the British Library

Acquisitions: Gina Almond
Development: Simone Dudziak and Julie Elliott
Set in 9.5/12 Palatino by TechBooks, New Delhi, India
Printed and bound by Replika Press Pvt. Ltd, India

For further information on Blackwell Publishing, visit our website:
www.blackwellcardiology.com

The publisher's policy is to use permanent paper from mills that operate a sustainable forestry policy, and which has been manufactured from pulp processed using acid-free and elementary chlorine-free practices. Furthermore, the publisher ensures that the text paper and cover board used have met acceptable environmental accreditation standards.

Notice: The indications and dosages of all drugs in this book have been recommended in the medical literature and conform to the practices of the general community. The medications described do not necessarily have specific approval by the Food and Drug Administration for use in the diseases and dosages for which they are recommended. The package insert for each drug should be consulted for use and dosage as approved by the FDA. Because standards for usage change, it is advisable to keep abreast of revised recommendations, particularly those concerning new drugs.

Contents

Foreword

Preexcitation syndromes have fascinated physicians for decades. Most of the interest is focused on the Wolff–Parkinson–White syndrome, which has been anatomically and pathophysiologically characterized in great detail. This book, titled *Variants of Ventricular Preexcitation: Recognition and Treatment*, by Eduardo Sternick and Hein Wellens offers insight into the many variant forms of preexcitation that are not well recognized.

After reviewing the history of these variants and discussing their pathological aspects, these authors have put together a compendium of well-described electrocardiographically and extremely well characterized electrophysiologically variant accessory pathways with which electrophysiologists still lack experience. The initial chapter reviewing the history and anatomy of the pathways is very useful in placing in perspective the differences between the pathologic and clinical aspects of these variant forms. A different classification of preexcitation syndromes is proposed, with the most important characteristic of the majority of these variants being decremental conduction. While the Wolff–Parkinson–White syndrome involves short atrioventricular bypass tracts with rapid conduction, the variants that have been described in this volume include short and long decrementally conducting atrioventricular bypass tracts and decrementally conducting atriofascicular bypass tracts. The outlyer in the group are the fasciculoventricular bypass tracts, which have no decremental properties and no participation in active reentrant arrhythmias but lead to curious electrocardiographic abnormalities that must be recognized by clinicians. Extensive discussions of the electrophysiological characteristics of all of these forms of preexcitation are well presented. A wealth of information exists in this text that can be found nowhere else. Examples of these variants and their electrophysiological features are clearly depicted and provide insights that cannot be found in any single source. The treatment of the decrementally conducting bypass tracts is described and is, as expected, primarily ablative. How to define the presence of these bypass tracts and distinguish them from others is and remains a very difficult but necessary test if one is to have a successful ablative therapy. The explanations of how to evaluate each of these forms of preexcitation in the laboratory and make the diagnosis correctly is a major feature of the text. In some ways, *Variants of Ventricular Preexcitation: Recognition and Treatment* provides a unique opportunity for general cardiologists and electrophysiologists to find in one text the intricacies of recognizing and treating a group of disorders that has intrigued physicians for more than 100 years.

Mark E. Josephson, MD
Chief, Cardiovascular Division
Beth Israel Deaconess Medical Center
Boston, USA

Acknowledgements

We would like to thank the important contributions made by the following people. Drs Luz-Maria Rodriguez and Carl Timmermans, University Hospital, Maastricht, The Netherlands; Dr Luiz Gerken, Biocor Instituto, Nova Lima, Brazil; Drs Fernando Cruz Filho and Márcio Fagundes, Instituto de Cardiologia Laranjeiras, Rio de Janeiro, Brazil; Drs Eduardo Sosa and Maurício Scanavacca, INCOR, São Paulo University, Brazil; Drs Gerard and Collette Guiraudon, London, Canada; Drs Michel Haissaguerre, Pierre Jais and Jacques Clementy, University Hospital, Bordeaux, France.

They helped us in many ways to accomplish our goal to write a book about the variants of pre-excitation.

A special word of thanks goes to Dr Mark Josephson. Not only because he was willing to write a foreword to our book, but also because he has been a fabulous teacher and role model for one of us, and an inspiring colleague and unique friend, during several decades, for the other!

Eduardo Back Sternick and Hein JJ Wellens

CHAPTER 1

Historical notes and classification of the variants of ventricular preexcitation

Almost 25 years ago, Gallagher *et al.* [1] stated that "the role of Mahaim fibers in the genesis of cardiac arrhythmias in man has been controversial since they were first described." The original description of these fibers was made by Ivan Mahaim in the late 1930s [2, 3] (Fig. 1.1).

He found a conducting tissue extending from the atrioventricular (AV) node to the ventricular myocardium. There are only a few articles dealing with anatomical studies of Mahaim fibers [3–8]. Early investigators found that Mahaim fibers were accessory connections taking off from the bundle of His and the fascicles (fasciculoventricular [FV] fibers) into the right ventricle or from the AV node (nodoventricular [NV] fibers) to the right ventricle or to the right bundle branch (nodofascicular [NF] fibers). Anderson *et al.* [9] proposed two varieties of NV fibers: one arising in the transitional zone and the other taking off from the deep, compact nodal portion of the AV junction. The NV concept was consistent with the findings published in the Gallagher series [1] series, wherein some patients had ventriculoatrial (VA) block during wide, complex tachycardia, proving that in those patients the atrium was not part of the reentrant circuit. Wellens [10] was the first to report the electrophysiological findings by using the technique of programmed electrical stimulation in a patient with an accessory pathway with decremental properties and long conduction times and assuming the pathway's relationship with the fibers described long ago by Mahaim. The term *nodofascicular* was used when the retrograde right bundle branch potential preceded the ventricular deflection, whereas the pathway was assumed to be *nodoventricular* when the retrograde His bundle deflection followed the beginning of the ventricular potential. The next step was the understanding of the functional significance and the anatomical–electrophysiological relationship of such pathways. An important observation was made in 1978 by Becker *et al.* [7] when they described an accessory AV node associated with a bundle of specialized fibers measuring 1 cm, coursing through the right ventricle, and mimicking a second AV conduction system located on the lateral tricuspid annulus. However, this finding did not change the mainstream concept of NV fibers at that time.

During the early 1980s, cardiologists started to refer patients with drug refractory tachycardias due to Mahaim fibers for surgical treatment. Although Gillette *et al.* [11] reported as early as 1982 a Mahaim fiber located on the anterior

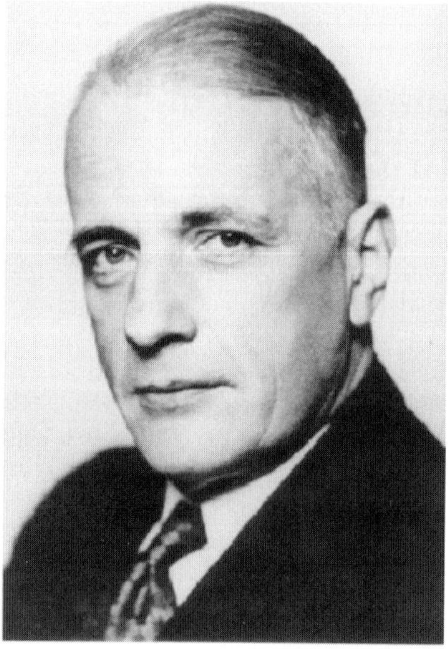

Figure 1.1 Ivan Mahaim (1897–1965). Born in Liège, Belgium, and educated in Lausanne, Switzerland, he was a fellow of Prof. Wenckebach in Vienna (1926). Mahaim wrote more than 100 papers, which were published in the leading journals of his time. His most influential works were his books on histological research concerning the connections of the bundle of His. This research was a resounding success in Europe in 1937 because it provided the basis for later electrophysiological discoveries. His last work, still a reference for musicians, was devoted to Beethoven's last quartets and published in 1964.

portion of the tricuspid ring, according to the concepts at that time, ablation of the AV node was considered to be the logical strategy for curative treatment of patients with NV/NF fibers. Some electrophysiologists introduced a new technique delivering high-energy current through a catheter to achieve ablation of the AV node to treat a patient with a Mahaim fiber. This technique resulted in complete AV block but persistent ventricular preexcitation [12]. The turning point came in 1988, when Klein *et al.* [13] decided to extensively freeze the AV node and the upper His bundle region of a 29-year-old man and discovered that preexcitation did not go away. This finding indicated to them that the accessory pathway was not connected with the AV node. In another patient the AV node was not damaged, but the decrementally conducting accessory pathway was successfully blocked by ice mapping at the right lateral aspect of the tricuspid annulus. Klein's manuscript was published in 1988. Shortly thereafter, Tchou *et al.* [14] published a paper titled "Atriofascicular Connection or a Nodoventricular Fiber? Electrophysiologic Elucidation of the Pathway and Associated Reentrant Circuit." In this elegant study the authors describe a simple maneuver to prove that such pathways are in fact inserting in the atrium and not in the A-V node. They showed that it was possible to advance ventricular depolarization during preexcited tachycardia by delivering late atrial premature beats during AV node refractoriness. In the following years, catheter ablation techniques shed more light on the subject. Discrete high-frequency potentials resembling the His bundle potential, considered the electrical activation of the atriofascicular pathway, were used as an effective target for ablation [(15, 16]. Observations during pharmacological interventions

[17], histological data [7, 8, 18, 19], electrophysiological maneuvers, and findings during radiofrequency catheter ablation, such as heat-induced automaticity while ablating at the atrial aspect of the annulus [22, 23]and also spontaneous automaticity [24], were presented as further evidence that the Mahaim fiber was composed of AV node-like tissue. Some authors [20] believed that an accessory AV node without a direct connection to the ventricle could be the substrate of atrial tachycardias mapped to the lateral tricuspid ring. They showed potentials preceding the P wave and decremental conduction between those potentials (M?) and the P wave and also the occurrence of automaticity during radiofrequency catheter ablation. NV/NF fibers are now considered a rare finding. Hluchy *et al.* [25]reported their presence in some patients with a narrow and regular QRS tachycardia with AV dissociation.

Recent reports using noncontact technologies for intracardiac mapping of atriofascicular pathways, such as the EnSite [26] and the LocaLisa system [27], have validated old data derived from open heart epicardial mapping and intracardiac catheter mapping [11, 13], suggesting that most of the decrementally conducting fibers are long structures connecting the right atrium to the anterior apical region of the right ventricle, close to or inserting into the distal part of the right bundle branch. There are a few reports of left-sided decrementally conducting accessory pathways, mostly decrementally conducting AV pathways connecting the left atrium to the left ventricle. Their distal end is usually mapped to the mitral annulus [28–30].

FV pathways [31] are anatomically different from atriofascicular pathways. They do not have long conduction times or decremental properties. Since they are infra-AV nodal structures connected to the His bundle or its fascicles, only the AV node shows decremental conduction. FV pathways play no role in clinical tachycardias. However, because its preexcitation pattern on the 12-lead electrocardiogram may resemble that of an anteroseptal accessory pathway [32], which is often associated with rapidly conducting bypass tracts, a misdiagnosis of a bypass tract should be avoided to prevent unnecessary damage to the AV node–His bundle conduction system by catheter ablation.

Critical analysis of the classification of preexcitation variants

The preexcitation syndromes were originally classified on the basis of their anatomical location and course and named according to the original investigators. This classification resulted in Mahaim, James, and Kent fibers. Later, such a description was considered inadequate because it did not fit the new electrophysiological or anatomical knowledge. In 1975 the European Study Group for Preexcitation [9] introduced a new classification based on the anatomical connections of the accessory pathways. However, the eponym Mahaim survived the changes proposed by the group. Why? It seems that the major issue here is the common electrophysiological finding of long and decremental conduction properties (AV node-like behavior) of such pathways, the so-called Mahaim physiology. We also need to emphasize that the eponym Mahaim

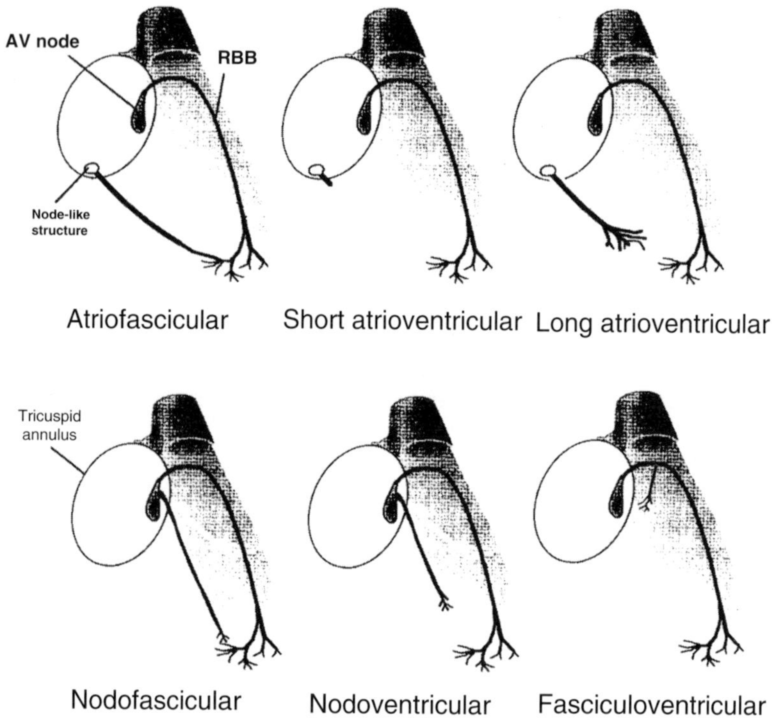

Figure 1.2 The different anatomical courses of preexcitation variants.

is already known to generations of arrhythmologists who witnessed the long and exciting process that took place until full understanding of the anatomical-functional relationship became possible. An updated anatomical classification of the preexcitation variants follows and is illustrated in Fig. 1.2.

Proximal insertion in the AV node–His bundle branch system:

1 NF bypass tract;
2 NV bypass tract;
3 FV pathway.

Proximal insertion in the atrium (right and left atrium):

1 Atriofascicular pathway;
2 short AV pathway with prolonged and decremental conduction;
3 long AV pathway with prolonged and decremental conduction.

References

1 Gallagher JJ, Smith WM, Kassell JH, *et al*. Role of Mahaim fibers in cardiac arrhythmias in man. *Circulation* 1981;64:176.

2 Luderitz B. Ivan Mahaim. *J Int Card Electrophysiol* 2003;8:155.

3 Mahaim I, Benatt A. Nouvelles recherches sur les connexions supérieures de la branche gauche du faisceau de His-Tawara avec cloison interventriculaire. *Cardiologia* 1938;1:61.

4 Mahaim I, Winston MR. Recherches d'anatomie comparée et de pathologie expérimentale sur le connexions hautes du faisceau de His-Tawara. *Cardiologia* 1941;5:189.

5 Lev M, Gibson S, Miller RA. Ebstein's disease with Wolff–Parkinson–White syndrome. *Am Heart J* 1955;49:724.

6 Lev M, Sodi-Palhares D, Friedlan C. A histopathologic study of the atrioventricular communications in a case of WPW with incomplete left bundle branch block. *Am Heart J* 1963;66:399.

7 Becker AE, Anderson RH, Durrer D, Wellens HJJ. The anatomical substrates of Wolff-Parkinson-White syndrome: a clinico-pathologic correlation in seven patients. *Circulation* 1978;57:870.

8 Anderson RH, Becker AE. Stanley Kent and accessory atrioventricular connections. *J Thoracic Cardiovasc Surg* 1981;81:649.

9 Anderson RH, Becker AE, Brechenmacher C, *et al.* Ventricular preexcitation. A proposed nomenclature for its substrates. *Eur J Cardiol* 1975;3:27.

10 Wellens HJJ. *Electrical Stimulation of the Heart in the Study and Treatment of Tachycardias.* Baltimore: University Park Press; 1971:97.

11 Gillette PC, Garson A, Cooley DA, *et al.* Prolonged and decremental anterograde conduction properties in right anterior accessory connections: wide QRS antidromic tachycardia of left bundle branch block pattern without Wolff–Parkinson–White configuration in sinus rhythm. *Am Heart J* 1982;103:66.

12 Bhandari A, Morady F, Shen EN, *et al.* Catheter-induced His bundle ablation in a patient with reentrant tachycardia associated with a nodoventricular tract. *J Am Coll Cardiol* 1984;4:611.

13 Klein GJ, Guiraudon GM, Kerr CR, *et al.* "Nodoventricular" accessory pathway: evidence for a distinct accessory atrioventricular pathway with atrioventricular node-like properties. *J Am Coll Cardiol* 1988;11:1035.

14 Tchou P, Lehmann MH, Jazayeri M, Akhtar M. Atriofascicular connection or a nodoventricular Mahaim fiber? Electrophysiologic elucidation of the pathway and associated reentrant circuit. *Circulation* 1988;77:837.

15 Brugada J, Martinez-Sanches J, Kuzmicic B, *et al.* Radiofrequency catheter ablation of atriofascicular accessory pathways guided by discrete electrical potentials recorded at the tricuspid annulus. *PACE* 1995;18:1388.

16 McClelland JH, Wang X, Beckman KJ, *et al.* Radiofrequency catheter ablation of right atriofascicular (Mahaim) accessory pathways guided by accessory pathway activation potentials. *Circulation* 1994;89:2655.

17 Ellenbogen KA, Rogers R, Old W. Pharmacological characterization of conduction over a Mahaim fiber: evidence for adenosine sensitive conduction. *Pacing Clin Electrophysiol* 1989;12:1396.

18 Guiraudon CM, Guiraudon GM, Klein GJ. Histologic evidence for an accessory atrioventricular pathway with AV-node-like morphology. *Circulation* 1988;78(suppl 2):40.

19 Epstein MR, Saul JP, Weindling SN, *et al.* Atrioventricular reciprocating tachycardia involving twin atrioventricular nodes in patients with complex congenital heart disease. *J Cardiovasc Electrophysiol* 2001;12:671.

20 Nogami A, Suguta M, Tomita T, *et al.* Novel form of atrial tachycardia originating at the atrioventricular annulus. *PACE* 1998;21:2691.

21 Gollob MB, Bharati S, Swerdlow CD. Accessory atrioventricular node with properties of a typical accessory pathway: anatomic-electrophysiologic correlation. *J Cardiovasc Electrophysiol* 2000;11:922.

22 Braun E, Siebbels J, Volkmer M, *et al.* Radiofrequency-induced preexcited automatic rhythm during ablation of accessory pathways with Mahaim-type preexcitation: does it predicts clinical outcome? *PACE* 1997;20(4, part 2):1121.
23 Sternick EB, Gerken LM, Vrandecic MO. Appraisal of "Mahaim" automatic tachycardia. *J Cardiovasc Electrophysiol* 2002;13:244.
24 Sternick EB, Timmermans C, Sosa E, *et al.* Automaticity in Mahaim fibers. *J Cardiovasc Electrophysiol* 2004;15:738.
25 Hluchy J, Schickel S, Jörger U, *et al.* Electrophysiologic characteristics and radiofrequency ablation of concealed nodofascicular and left anterograde atriofascicular pathways. *J Cardiovasc Electrophysiol* 2000;11:211.
26 Fung WHJ, Chan HCK, Chan WWL, Sanderson JE. Ablation of the Mahaim pathway guided by noncontact mapping. *J Cardiovasc Electrophysiol* 2002;13:1064.
27 Tan HL, Wittkampf FHM, Nakagawa H, Derksen R. Atriofascicular accessory pathway. *J Cardiovasc Electrophysiol* 2004;15:118.
28 Goldberger JJ, Pederson DN, Damle RS, *et al.* Antidromic tachycardia utilizing decremental, latent accessory atrioventricular fibers: differentiation from adenosine-sensitive ventricular tachycardia. *J Am Coll Cardiol* 1994;24:732.
29 Johnson CT, Brooks C, Jaramillo J, *et al.* Left free-wall, decrementally conducting atrioventricular (Mahaim) fiber: diagnosis at electrophysiologic study and radiofrequency catheter ablation guided by direct recording of a Mahaim potential. *PACE* 1997;20:2486
30 Tada H, Nogami A, Naito S, *et al.* Left posteroseptal Mahaim fiber associated with marked longitudinal dissociation. *PACE* 1999;22:1696.
31 Sternick EB, Gerken LM, Vrandecic M, Wellens HJJ. Fasciculoventricular pathways: clinical and electrophysiologic characteristics of a variant of preexcitation. *J Cardiovasc Electrophysiol* 2003;14:1057.
32 Sternick EB, Rodriguez LM, Gerken LM, Wellens HJJ. The electrocardiogram of patients with fasciculoventricular pathways. A comparative study with patients with anteroseptal and midseptal accessory pathways. *Heart Rhythm* 2005;2:1.

CHAPTER 2

The anatomy of decrementally conducting fibers

In the early 1940s, Ivan Mahaim described the presence of "fines hautes connexions" (delicate proximal connections), also called paraspecific fibers, which connect the central part of the AV node and the penetrating bundle of His directly to the ventricle [1, 2]. They were considered to be remnants of the embryonic anlagen of the conducting tissues. Indeed, these "remnants" can be identified in infantile, adolescent, and adult hearts, be it in a decreasing or increasing frequency.

Mahaim concluded that these fibers may serve as septal conduction pathways – that is, as an alternative to the bundle branch–Purkinje system, but with a wide spectrum of variability in dimensions and locations. Mahaim attempted to demonstrate their functional role by showing experimentally that sequential cutting of these connections modified the surface electrocardiogram (ECG).

Anderson and Becker [3] studied an embryonic human heart in which multiple atrioventricular (AV) connections, as described by Mahaim, were present; but during electrical stimulation of the atrium, AV conduction occurred over the normal conduction system. However, Lev *et al.* studied specimens in which the fibers were considered to be of conductive significance [4]. In 1971 Wellens [5] reported the electrophysiological findings in a young boy having paroxysmal tachycardia caused by an accessory pathway with decremental properties. This finding renewed interest in the anatomical-functional relationship of Mahaim fibers.

A few years thereafter, Anderson *et al.* [6] classified the Mahaim connections as nodoventricular (NV) fibers, taking off from the compact node and fasciculoventricular (FV) connections originating more distally in the AV junctional area.

There is a case report correlating the presence of an NV fiber with the occurrence of paroxysmal tachycardias in an 11-year-old boy who had a cardiac arrest while tobogganing. He was found in ventricular fibrillation and was resuscitated, but developed a persistent vegetative state for 3 years and eventually died [7]. At autopsy, the complete AV junction, including the left and the right parietal zone as well as the septal junctional zone, was removed for histological studies. It was found that a discrete tract of specialized conduction cells was present, obliquely traversing through connective tissues becoming continuous with myocardial cells at the crest of the ventricular septum. The calculated length and width of the bundle were 8 and 1 mm, respectively.

Becker *et al.* [8] made another important observation in 1978, when they described an accessory AV node associated with a bundle of specialized fibers (1 cm long) coursing through the right ventricle, and mimicking a second atrioventricular conduction system located on the lateral tricuspid annulus. However, this finding at that time did not challenge the prevailing concept that Mahaim fibers were NV connections.

During the early 1980s, patients with drug refractory tachycardias due to Mahaim fibers were referred for surgical treatment. Although Gillette *et al.* [9] reported as early as 1982 a Mahaim fiber located on the anterior portion of the tricuspid ring, according to the concept at that point in time, ablation of the AV node was considered to be the logical strategy for curative treatment of patients with NV fibers. However, when Bhandari *et al.* [10] attempted to treat a patient with a Mahaim fiber by delivering high-energy current through a catheter to achieve ablation of the A-V node complete AV block ensued while ventricular preexcitation persisted [10]. In 1988, Dr. Guiraudon and his associates [11] operated upon a patient with a decrementally conducting accessory pathway by freezing the A-V node and upper His bundle region. However ventricular preexcitation did not disappear. That finding indicated to them that the accessory pathway was not connected with the A-V node. In their next patient the Mahaim fiber was successfully ablated while AV node conduction was preserved.

During open-heart surgery of at least three patients with decrementally conducting accessory pathways, Dr Gerard Guiraudon, before applying cryoablation, excised a fragment of tissue from the site where the Mahaim fiber was mapped and had it examined by the pathologist Dr Colette Guiraudon. According to Dr Gerard Guiraudon, Dr Colette Guiraudon came to him after examining the microscopy of the biopsy specimens and asked why he was doing biopsies of the AV node in such patients!

Guiraudon *et al.* [12] presented their findings at the American Heart Association Meeting in 1988, and they generously allowed us to publish some examples in this chapter (see Plates 2.1 & 2.2, *facing p. 22*).

The observations mentioned earlier lead to the conclusion that "true Mahaim fibers" consisting of NV (or nodofascicular [NF]) fibers are rare and that "pseudo Mahaim fibers," mainly represented by the atriofascicular connections are more common.

To make matters even more complex, we recently learned that not all accessory AV nodes have decremental conduction. Gollob *et al.* reported a patient with an accessory AV node having the clinical picture of a rapidly conducting accessory pathway [13].

Short AV decrementally conducting fibers

The short AV Mahaim fibers are another variety of decrementally conducting fibers connecting the atrium to the ventricular myocardium. There is no morphological information available, but electrophysiological findings [14] suggest that this variety is an electrophysiologically heterogeneous group of fibers, some of which probably have an accessory AV node, without a long bundle, connecting with the ventricular musculature at the annulus, and others probably consisting of regular myocardial fibers. In the latter situation, decremental conduction can be explained by fiber tortuosity with anisotropic conduction, as in the case reported by Critelli *et al.* [15]. In one patient, Haissaguerre [16] reported the development of decremental conduction after a radiofrequency current ablation attempt of a rapidly conducting accessory pathway.

Another possibility could be the presence of an accessory pathway in glycogen storage disease, such as that caused by a mutant *PRKAG2* gene. According to Gollob *et al.*, who reported the association of familial Wolff–Parkinson–White (WPW) syndrome and left ventricular hypertrophy due to *PRKAG2* mutation, there was a high incidence (5 patients) of decrementally conducting accessory pathways among the 8 patients undergoing an electrophysiological evaluation [17].

Left-sided decrementally conducting fibers

The anatomical basis for the presence of a left-sided Mahaim fiber comes from the work of Anderson *et al.* [18]. In 15 % of normal adult hearts, they found AV node-like structures around the tricuspid annulus and the posterior margin of the mitral annulus. These were considered to be remnants of the specialized AV ring tissue from which the normal conduction system develops. Lev *et al.* [3] described Mahaim fibers (FV pathways) taking off from the His bundle and connecting to both the right and the left side of the septum on autopsy of a 54-year-old woman who, however, only had ECG evidence of a right-sided AV pathway.

Left-sided FV pathway

One of our 8 cases, with an ECG and electrophysiological evidence, had an FV pathway connected to the left side of the interventricular septum [19].

Left-sided NV pathway

In 1987 Abbott *et al.* [20] reported on two patients with coexistent Kent and Mahaim accessory connections. Although no definite conclusion could be reached, the Mahaim fibers were described as NV connections inserting in or near the left posterior fascicle.

Left-sided AV pathway

A few years later, Yamabe *et al.* [21] reported on a 44-year-old patient with palpitations due to an orthodromic tachycardia by using a concealed left lateral bypass tract for retrograde conduction. The QRS complexes showed a variable degree of a right bundle branch block configuration (with short HV intervals) caused by anterograde conduction over a decremental pathway probably connecting to the left posterior fascicle.

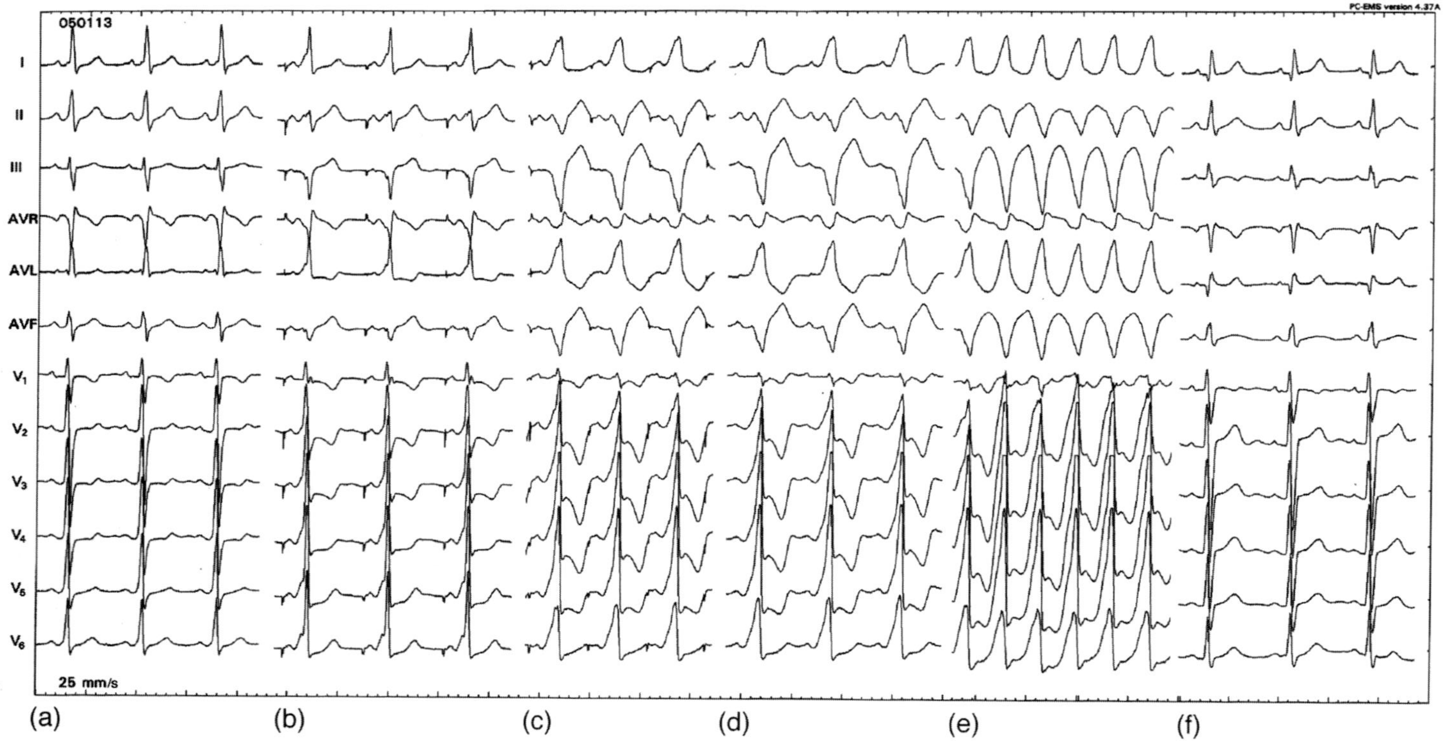

Figure 2.1 A 12-lead ECG. (a) Sinus rhythm showing minimal preexcitation; (b) atrial pacing (450 ms), showing that the QRS complex is more preexcited; (c) atrial pacing at a shorter cycle length (350 ms), showing maximal preexcitation; (d) 12 mg of adenosine causes block in the AV node but not at the accessory fiber; (e) AVNRT with bystander anterograde conduction over the short AV Mahaim fiber; (f) sinus rhythm after catheter ablation of the left midseptal Mahaim fiber. Courtesy of Dr Fernando ES Cruz, and Dr Márcio Fagundes.

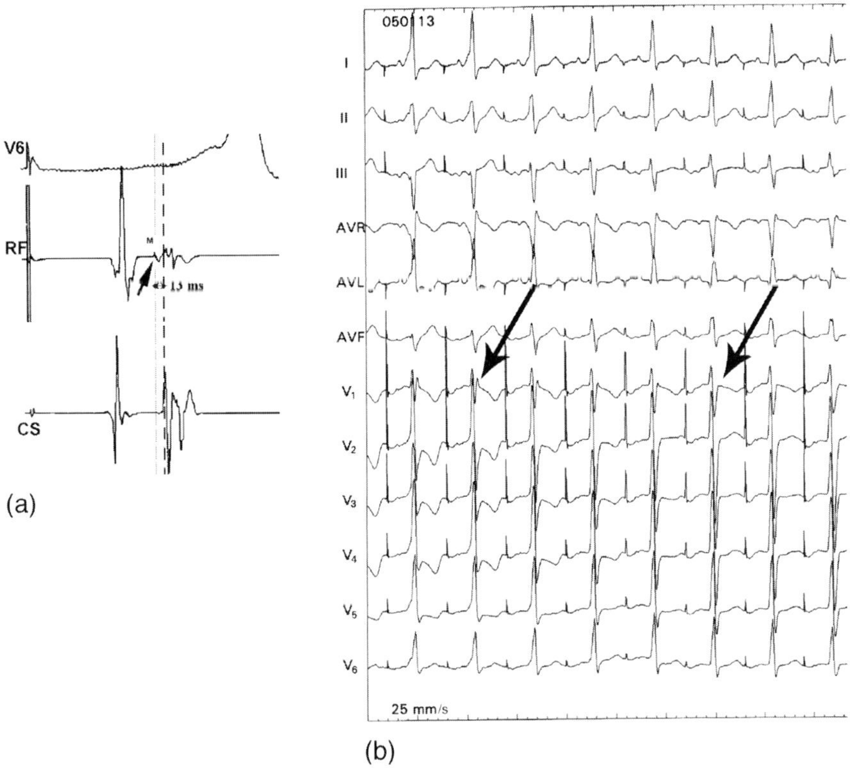

Figure 2.2 (a) An accessory pathway potential (M potential) was recorded at the mitral annulus, 13 ms earlier than the local ventricular potential. (b) A 12-lead ECG: RF current was delivered during atrial pacing. There was no automaticity arising in the left-sided, short, decrementally conducting accessory pathway. Note the terminal r' in V1, which disappears after successful ablation of the decrementally conducting fiber (arrows). Courtesy of Dr Fernando ES Cruz, and Dr Márcio Fagundes.

However, solid data about a left-sided decrementally conducting AV fiber were first provided in 1994 by Goldberger *et al.* [22], who successfully ablated a decrementally conducting left posteroseptal AV pathway. The antidromic tachycardia showed a right bundle branch block-like configuration and a left superior QRS axis. Activation mapping during tachycardia located the decrementally conducting fiber at the mitral annulus.

Johnson *et al.* [23] described a 64-year-old woman with a WPW syndrome. She had a rapidly conducting right-sided AV pathway and a decrementally conducting left-sided free-wall AV pathway. Successful catheter ablation of the second fiber was accomplished by targeting an M potential found at the lateral mitral annulus during tachycardia. Tada *et al.* [24] also reported a patient who underwent radiofrequency catheter ablation of a left posteroseptal AV decrementally conducting fiber. The earliest ventricular activation was recorded at the mitral annulus with a QS-like unipolar recording, with a local

AV conduction time of 62 milliseconds. Most left-sided short AV decrementally conducting accessory pathways lack AV node-like characteristics such as sensitivity to intravenous adenosine and absence of heat-induced automaticity during radiofrequency catheter ablation. Dr Cruz recently ablated one patient having recurrent episodes of an AV nodal reentry tachycardia (AVNRT) with occasional bystander conduction over a left-sided short AV Mahaim fiber. He kindly allowed us to publish a figure from the study of this patient (Figs 2.1 & 2.2).

Left-sided Atriofascicular pathway

Hluchy *et al.* [25] studied a 31-year-old woman who had recurrent symptomatic tachycardia with a right bundle branch block pattern and a left superior QRS axis. A long, left posteroseptal atriofascicular pathway connected with the left bundle branch was suggested by the following findings: a His bundle potential inside the QRS during RBBB-shaped tachycardia; evidence of an atrial origin of the AP by showing advancement of ventricular activation by a late left atrial premature beat during antidromic tachycardia; recording of an M potential at both the atrial and ventricular insertion; catheter-induced transient mechanical block; and successful catheter ablation at the atrial insertion site.

From these observations we have learned that the majority of the left-sided Mahaim fibers seem to be short, decrementally conducting AV pathways connecting the left atrium with the left ventricle at the mitral annulus, mostly in the posteroseptal area.

References

1 Mahaim I, Winston MR. Recherches d'anatomie compare et de pathologie expérimentale sur les connexions hautes du faisceau de His-Tawara. *Cardiologia* 1941;5:189.

2 Mahaim I. Kent's fibers and the AV paraspecific conduction through the upper connection of the bundle of His-Tawara. *Am Heart J* 1947;33:651.

3 Anderson RH, Becker AE. Morphology of the human atrioventricular junctional area. In: Wellens HJJ, Lie KI, Janse MJ, eds. *The Conduction System of the Heart: Structure, Functions and Clinical Implications*. Leiden, the Netherlands: HE Stenfert Kroese BV; 1976:261.

4 Lev M, Fox SM, Bharati S, *et al.* Mahaim and James fibers as a basis for a unique variety of pre-excitation. *Am J Cardiol* 1975;35:152.

5 Wellens HJJ. *Electrical Stimulation of the Heart in the Study and Treatment of Tachycardias.* Baltimore: University Park Press; 1971:97.

6 Anderson RH, Becker AE, Brechenmacher C, Davies MJ, Rossi L. Ventricular pre-excitation. A proposed nomenclature for its substrates. *Eur J Cardiol* 1975;3:27.

7 Gmeiner R, Keung C, Hammer I, Becker AE. Tachycardia caused by an accessory nodoventricular tract: a clinico-pathologic correlation. *Eur Heart J* 1984;5:233.

8 Becker AE, Anderson RH, Durrer D, Wellens HJJ. The anatomical substrates of Wolff–Parkinson–White syndrome: a clinico-pathologic correlation in seven patients. *Circulation* 1978;57:870.

9 Gillette PC, Garson A, Cooley DA, *et al.* Prolonged and decremental anterograde conduction properties in right anterior accessory connections: wide QRS antidromic tachycardia of left bundle branch block pattern without Wolff–Parkinson–White configuration in sinus rhythm. *Am Heart J* 1982;103:66.
10 Bhandari A, Morady F, Shen EN, *et al.* Catheter-induced His bundle ablation in a patient with reentrant tachycardia associated with a nodoventricular tract. *J Am Coll Cardiol* 1984;4:611.
11 Klein GJ, Guiraudon GM, Kerr CR, *et al.* "Nodoventricular" accessory pathway: evidence for a distinct accessory atrioventricular pathway with atrioventricular node-like properties. *J Am Coll Cardiol* 1988;11:1035.
12 Guiraudon CM, Guiraudon GM, Klein GJ. Histologic evidence for an accessory atrioventricular pathway with AV-node-like morphology. *Circulation* 1988;78(suppl 2):40.
13 Gollob M, Bharati S, Swerdlow CD. Accessory atrioventricular node with properties of a typical accessory pathway: anatomic-electrophysiologic correlation. *J Cardiovasc Electrophysiol* 2000;11:922.
14 Sternick EB, Fagundes M, Cruz Filho FE, *et al.* Short atrioventricular Mahaim fiber: observations on their clinical, eletrocardiographic and electrophysiologic profile. *J Cardiovasc Electrophysiol* 2005;16:127.
15 Critelli G, Perticone F, Coltorti F, *et al.* Antegrade slow bypass conduction after closed-chest ablation of the His bundle in permanent junctional reciprocating tachycardia. *Circulation* 1983;67:687.
16 Haissaguerre M, Cauchemez B, Marcus F, *et al.* Characteristics of the ventricular insertion sites of accessory pathways with anterograde decremental conduction properties. *Circulation* 1995;91:1077.
17 Gollob M, Green MS, Tang ASL, *et al.* Identification of a gene responsible for familial Wolff–Parkinson–White syndrome. *N Engl J Med* 2001;344:1823.
18 Anderson RH, Davies MJ, Becker AE. Atrioventricular ring specialized tissue in the normal heart. *Eur J Cardiol* 1974;2:219.
19 Sternick EB, Rodriguez LM, Gerken LM, Wellens HJJ. The electrocardiogram of patients with fasciculoventricular pathways. A comparative study with patients with anteroseptal and midseptal accessory pathways. *Heart Rhythm* 2005;2:1.
20 Abbott JA, Scheinman MM, Morady F, *et al.* Coexistent Mahaim and Kent accessory connections: diagnostic and therapeutic implications. *J Am Coll Cardiol* 1987;10:364.
21 Yamabe H, Okumura K, Minoda K, Yasue H. Nodoventricular Mahaim fiber connecting to the left ventricle. *Am Heart J* 1991;122:232.
22 Goldberger JJ, Pederson DN, Damle RS, *et al.* Antidromic tachycardia utilizing decremental, latent accessory atrioventricular fibers: differentiation from adenosine-sensitive ventricular tachycardia. *J Am Coll Cardiol* 1994;24:732.
23 Johnson CT, Brooks C, Jaramillo J, *et al.* Left free-wall, decrementally conducting atrioventricular (Mahaim) fiber: diagnosis at electrophysiologic study and radiofrequency catheter ablation guided by direct recording of a Mahaim potential. *PACE* 1997;20:2486.
24 Tada H, Nogami A, Naito S, *et al.* Left posteroseptal Mahaim fiber associated with marked longitudinal dissociation. *PACE* 1999;22:1696.
25 Hluchy J, Schickel S, Jorger U, *et al.* Electrophysiologic characteristics and radiofrequency ablation of concealed nodofascicular and left anterograde atriofascicular pathways. *J Cardiovasc Electrophysiol* 2000;11:211.

CHAPTER 3

Atriofascicular pathways and decrementally conducting long atrioventricular pathways

Introduction

There has been extensive debate concerning the anatomic structure [1–4], location [5–7], related arrhythmias [8, 9], electrophysiological properties [10–12], ablative techniques [13, 14], and automaticity [15] of accessory pathways with long and decremental anterograde conduction. Less attention has been given to the 12-lead electrocardiogram (ECG), especially to the ECG during sinus rhythm. The latter is considered to be normal in the majority of patients with atriofascicular pathways and patients with long atrioventricular (AV) decrementally conducting accessory pathways. Minimal preexcitation is reported to occur from 0 to 30% [13, 14, 16, 17], and apart from the absence of q waves in the left precordial leads [18], no specific QRS pattern has been described. We have studied a large cohort of patients with decrementally conducting fibers in order to assess the ECG findings during sinus rhythm and tachycardia [19], to appraise the current criteria in the differential diagnosis of patients with a left bundle branch block (LBBB)-shaped tachycardia [20], and a review of the cardiac arrhythmias occurring in the setting of an atriofascicular pathway [21].

The ECG during sinus rhythm and tachycardia

We retrospectively analyzed 12-lead ECGs from 38 patients having anterograde conduction over accessory pathways with long conduction times and decremental properties both during sinus rhythm and during tachycardia. Five patients also had anterograde rapidly conducting accessory pathways and were excluded from the study.

Definition of terms

We use the eponym Mahaim fibers in this study as a synonym of accessory pathways with long and decremental properties with a long anatomic course, either atriofascicular pathways (30 patients) or AV pathways (3 patients).

There were 20 female patients and 13 male patients, with a mean age of 24 ± 10 (range 8 to 52) years. All patients were referred for an electrophysiological assessment of a preexcited tachycardia. Preexcited AV nodal reentrant tachycardia (AVNRT) using a Mahaim fiber as a bystander was present in 1 patient.

One patient had atrial fibrillation with preexcited QRS complexes, and 2 patients were referred because of repetitive episodes of nonsustained tachycardia caused by automaticity arising in the Mahaim fiber [9] (Table 3.1). Ebstein's disease was diagnosed in 4 patients. The atrial insertion of the Mahaim fiber was located by the recording of a discrete accessory pathway potential in 28 patients and by assessing the shortest AV interval during atrial pacing at different sites around the tricuspid annulus in 5 patients. All patients underwent successful surgical ($n = 2$) or radiofrequency (RF) catheter ablation ($n = 31$). RF ablation

Table 3.1 Clinical data.

n	*Sex*	*Age*	*Site-TA*	*Arrhythmia*	*Ebstein*	*CBT*	*Therapy S/RF_p/RF-dis*
1	F	31	L	Antidromic AVRT/Mahaim			S
2	F	32	L	Antidromic AVRT/Mahaim AVNRT			RF_p
3	F	19	PL	Antidromic AVRT/Mahaim	Yes		RF_p
4	F	21	PL	Antidromic AVRT/Mahaim	Yes	RPS	RF_p
				Ortodromic AVRT			RF_p
5	M	52	PL	Preexcited atrial fibrillation			RF_p
6	M	21	L	Antidromic AVRT/Mahaim			RF_p
7	F	23	L	Antidromic AVRT/Mahaim			RF_p
8	F	19	A	Antidromic AVRT/Mahaim			RF_p
9	F	23	L	Antidromic AVRT/Mahaim			RF_p
10	F	25	PL	Antidromic AVRT/Mahaim			RF_p
11	M	35	L	Antidromic AVRT/Mahaim			RF_p
12	F	42	L	Antidromic AVRT/Mahaim			RF_p
13	F	23	L	Antidromic AVRT/Mahaim			RF_p
14	F	8	AL	Mahaim automaticity			RF_p
15	M	30	PL	Antidromic AVRT/Mahaim			RF_p
16	F	27	L	Antidromic AVRT/Mahaim			RF_p
17	F	19	L	Antidromic AVRT/Mahaim			RF_p
18	M	12	MS	Mahaim automaticity			RF_p
19	F	39	L	Antidromic AVRT/Mahaim			RF_p
20	F	15	AL	AVNRT+Mahaim bystander			RF_p
21	M	13	L	Antidromic AVRT/Mahaim			RF_p
22	M	15	A	Antidromic AVRT/Mahaim			RF_p
23	F	25	L	Antidromic AVRT/Mahaim			RF_p
24	M	18	L	Antidromic AVRT/Mahaim			RF_p
25	F	45	L	Antidromic AVRT/Mahaim			RF_p
26	M	24	L	Antidromic AVRT/Mahaim			RF-dis
27	M	11	L	Antidromic AVRT/Mahaim	Yes		S
28	M	26	L	Antidromic AVRT/Mahaim	Yes	LL	RF-dis
29	M	25	A	Antidromic AVRT/Mahaim			RF-dis
30	F	26	P	Antidromic AVRT/Mahaim			RF-dis
31	F	31	L	Antidromic AVRT/Mahaim			RF-dis
32	F	22	L	Antidromic AVRT/Mahaim			RF_p
33	M	17	P	Antidromic AVRT/Mahaim			RF_p

AL, right anterolateral; AVRT/Mahaim, reentrant tachycardia with AV conduction over a Mahaim fiber; CBT, concealed bypass tract; L, right lateral; LL, left lateral; MS, right midseptal; P, posterior; PL, right posterolateral; RPS, right posteroseptal; Site, site of ablation of the Mahaim fiber at the tricuspid annulus (TA); S/RFp/RF-dis, surgery/radiofrequency catheter ablation at the atrial/ventricular insertion.

was guided by discrete potentials at the tricuspid annulus (28 patients) and by right ventricular (RV) pace mapping (5 patients).

We also analyzed the 12-lead ECG during sinus rhythm in 200 individuals with palpitations and without structural heart disease matched for age and gender as a control group.

Definitions of the QRS patterns

ECGs were examined by two different observers with a magnified lens, and a third observer decided when there was a mismatch classification. The following QRS patterns were found: r/rS/RS/Rs/rsR′/rsr′/R/qR/QR/QS/qRs/qRS. Very low voltage QRS complexes (<0.3 millivolts) were depicted as small letters (r, rs, or rsr′). A QRS complex with a higher voltage was depicted according to the ratio between the positive (R, r) and the negative waves (q, Q, S, and s). For example, an RS complex is defined as the presence of a QRS complex showing an initially positive deflection followed by a negative deflection of even magnitude. Likewise, an Rs pattern means a QRS complex (>0.3 mV) with an initial positive deflection followed by a smaller negative one. A septal q wave is defined as a q wave in surface leads I, aVL, and V_6, with an amplitude less than 25% of the R wave and a width less than 0.04 seconds.

Statistical analysis

Values are given as mean ± standard deviation. The significance of differences ($p < 0.05$) between groups of clinical, electrocardiographic, or electrophysiological parameters was assessed by Student's t test or Fisher's exact test.

Results

Preablation 12-lead ECG findings

Minimal preexcitation, defined as subtle abnormalities suggesting the presence of preexcitation, with a QRS complex width within the normal range (<0.12 s) but with a short HV interval (<35 ms), was present during sinus rhythm in 24 patients (72%). The PR interval was not significantly different when comparing patients with (125 ± 21 ms) and without (132 ± 9 ms) minimal preexcitation ($p = \text{ns}$).

We found two patterns of the QRS complex (Fig. 3.1) during sinus rhythm, the most common one being an rS configuration in lead III. This was found in 20 patients. The other pattern in lead III, an rsR′, was found in 2 patients. In the presence of an rS pattern in lead III, no q wave was found in lead I in 15 patients (and in lead V_6 in 8 patients). Minimal preexcitation manifest with absence of a q wave in lead I (without an rS in lead III) was seen in only 2 patients (patients 8 and 16, Table 3.2).

In 3 patients, minimal preexcitation was not always manifest, as documented by 12-lead ECGs taken on different days. Variability of minimal preexcitation in the same ECG was seen in 2 patients (Fig. 3.2).

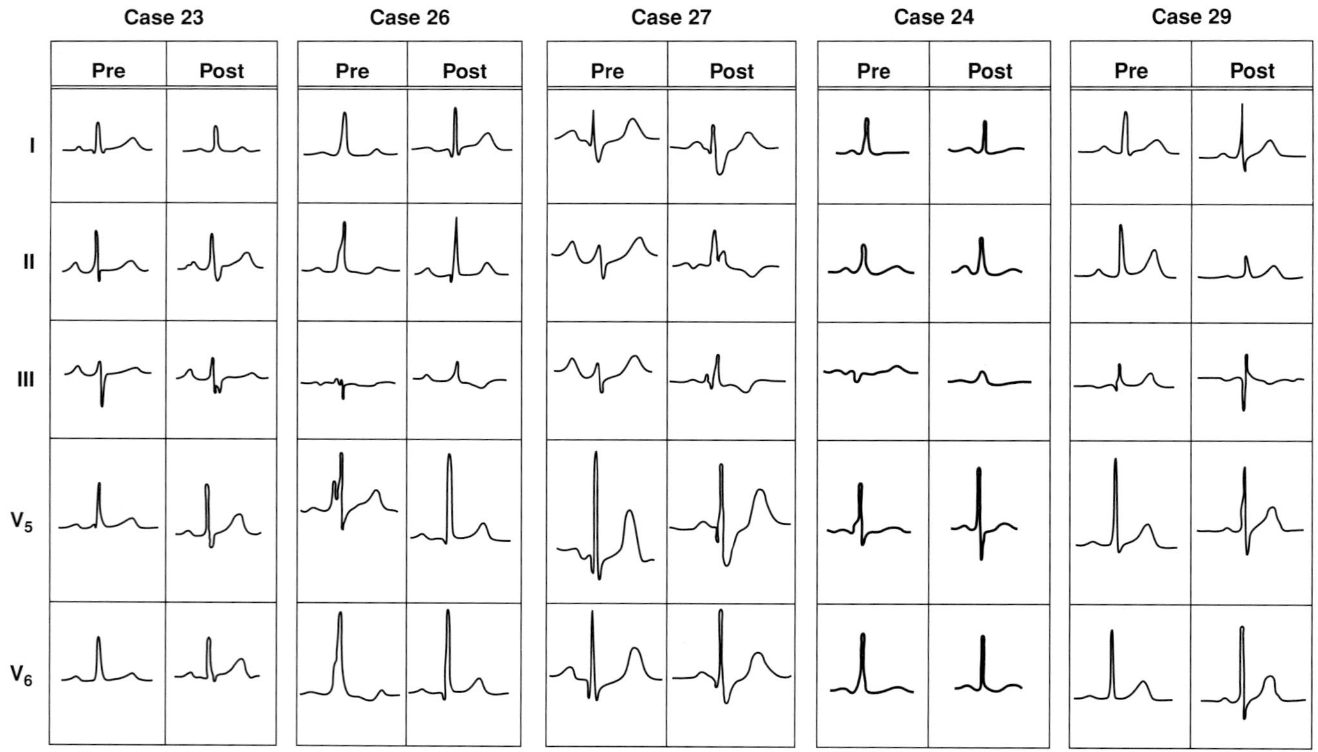

Figure 3.1 A 5-lead ECG during sinus rhythm with the preablation ECG showing the rS pattern in four cases and rsR' in 1 patient. The postablation ECG shows a clear change in QRS configuration.

Table 3.2 Electrocardiographic data of Mahaim fibers.

	Before Mahaim ablation									After ablation			
	Sinus rhythm						Tachycardia			Sinus rhythm			
n	*ECG BBB*	*PR*	*QRS width*	*Lead III pre*	*q-I pre*	*q-V6 pre*	*Lead III*	*Axis*	*QRS width*	*ECG BBB*	*Lead III post*	*q-I post*	*q-V6 post*
1		**0.13**	**0.11**	**rS**	No	No	rS	0	120		qR	No	Yes
2		**0.11**	**0.11**	**rS**	No	No	rS	−30	130		rs	No	No
3*		**0.12**	**0.08**	**rS**	No	No	rS	−45	140		qR	No	No
4*		0.14	0.08	qRs	No	No	rS	−45	130	RBB	qR	No	No
5		**0.12**	**0.09**	**rS**	No	No	rS	−45	130		rs	No	No
6		0.12	0.09	qR	No	No	rS	−30	120		qR	No	No
7		**0.11**	**0.08**	**rS**	No	No	rS	−15	120		qR	No	Yes
8		**0.13**	**0.08**	**qR**	Yes	No	R	−60	130		qR	No	Yes
9		**0.10**	**0.09**	**rS**	Yes	Yes	rS	−45	130		RS	No	Yes
10		**0.12**	**0.1**	**rS**	No	No	rS	−60	120		qR	Yes	Yes
11		**0.14**	**0.09**	**rS**	Yes	No	rS	15	120		rsr’	Yes	Yes
12		**0.11**	**0.1**	**rS**	No	No	rS	−30	130		qR	No	No
13		**0.13**	**0.12**	**rS**	No	Yes	rS	−30	120		qR	No	Yes
14		**0.14**	**0.09**	**rS**	No	No	rSr’	0	120		qR	No	No
15		**0.15**	**0.09**	**rS**	Yes	Yes	rS	−60	120		qR	No	No
16		**0.15**	**0.08**	**qR**	No	No	rS	−45	120		qR	No	Yes
17		0.14	0.08	qR	No	Yes	rS	−30	120		qR	No	Yes
18		**0.10**	**0.11**	**rS**	No	No	rS	−60	120		qR	No	Yes
19	LAD	0.13	0.11	rS*	Yes	No	rS	−45	120	LAD	rS	Yes	No
20		**0.12**	**0.1**	**rS**	No	No	rS	−45	130		qR	Yes	Yes
21		0.14	0.08	qR	No	Yes	rS	0	130		qR	No	Yes
22		0.12	0.09	qR	Yes	Yes	R	−60	130	RBB	qR	Yes	Yes
23		**0.12**	**0.1**	**rS**	No	No	rs	−30	120		qR	No	Yes
24		**0.11**	**0.1**	**rS**	No	No	rS	−30	130		qR	Yes	Yes
25	iRBB	**0.20**	**0.09**	**rS**	No	No	rS	−30	120	iRBB	qR	No	No
26		**0.10**	**0.1**	**rS**	No	No	rS	0	120		qR	Yes	Yes
27*	iRBB	**0.12**	**0.1**	**rS**	Yes	Yes	rS	−30	140	RBB	rsR’	Yes	Yes
28*		**0.12**	**0.1**	**rS**	Yes	Yes	rS	−75	120		qR	Yes	Yes
29		**0.12**	**0.09**	**rsR’**	No	No	RS	−15	140		QR	No	No
30		0.14	0.08	qR	No	No	rS	−60	120		qR	No	No
31		0.12	0.09	qR	No	No	rS	−60	120		qR	No	No
32		0.14	0.08	qR	Yes	Yes	rS	−30	140		qR	Yes	Yes
33		**0.14**	**0.09**	**rsR’**	No	No	rS	−30	140	RBB	qR	No	No

AP, accessory pathway. BBB, bundle branch block. Bold characters indicates patients with minimal preexcitation; *n**, patient with Ebstein's disease; PR, PR interval; pre/post, pre- or post-RF ablation.

Intracavitary signals, Mahaim potential recording and right bundle and His bundle electrogram

We found that the AM (atrium-proximal Mahaim potential, interval) I was always 20–40 milliseconds shorter than the AH interval in patients with minimal preexcitation. In patients without preexcitation the AH interval was shorter than the AM interval.

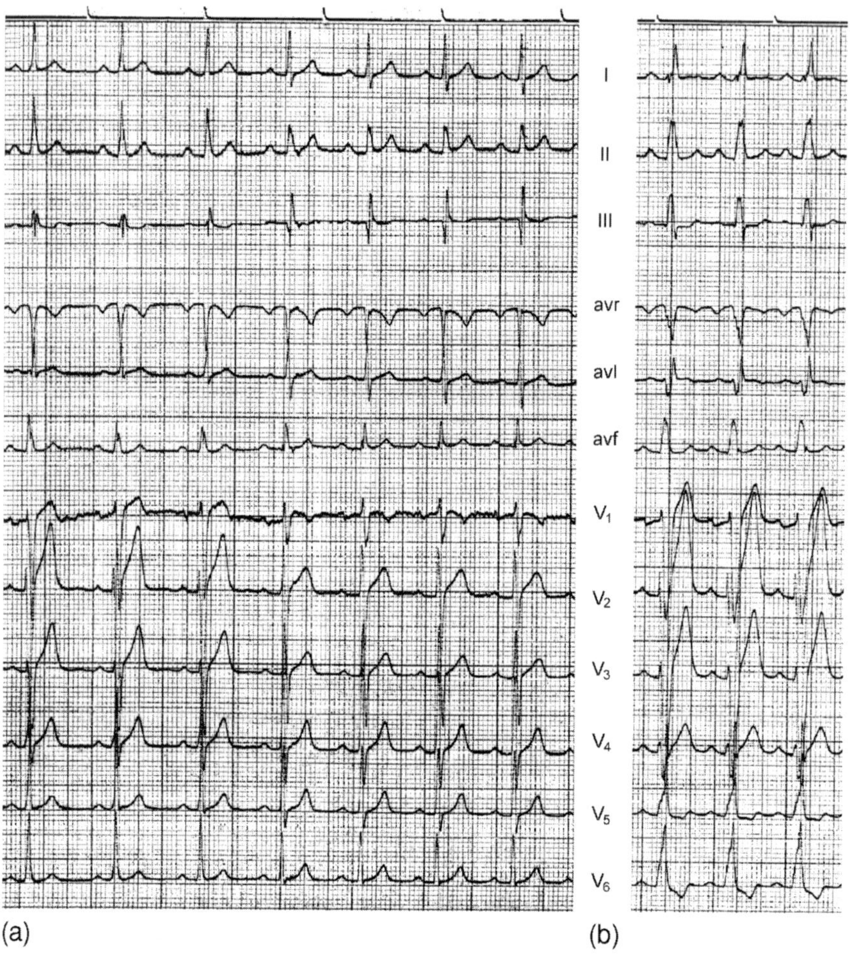

Figure 3.2 (a) ECG shows minimal preexcitation (rsR' pattern in lead III) only in the first 3 QRS complexes. (b) ECG after intravenous verapamil shows sinus rhythm with AV conduction over the Mahaim fiber with a long PR interval and overt preexcitation.

ECG during tachycardia

We analyzed 29 patients with a circus movement tachycardia with anterograde conduction over the Mahaim fiber, one AVNRT with bystander Mahaim conduction, one with atrial fibrillation with anterograde conduction over the Mahaim fiber, and two automatic tachycardias arising in the Mahaim fiber. During circus movement tachycardia the cycle length ranged from 430–250 milliseconds. QRS width during tachycardia (Table 3.2) varied from 120–140 milliseconds. All patients had a monophasic R wave in lead I, and 30 out of 33 patients had an rS in V_1 during tachycardia (3 patients had a QS in V_1).

Comparison between the ECG during sinus rhythm and during tachycardia with anterograde conduction over the Mahaim fiber

In all 20 patients with an rS pattern in lead III, we found a negative QRS complex in the same lead (either an rS or a QS pattern) during tachycardia (Fig. 3.3). Also the patient with atrial fibrillation showed a negative QRS complex. There were 9 patients without the rS pattern in lead III during sinus rhythm, which showed left-axis deviation during tachycardia. Three patients showed concordance between absence of an rS pattern during sinus rhythm and their tachycardia QRS pattern (all three patients had an anterior Mahaim) (Fig. 3.4).

Postablation 12-lead ECG

In the 24 patients showing minimal preexcitation in their 12-lead ECG, six patterns were observed in lead III during sinus rhythm after Mahaim ablation. The most common QRS configuration was a qR or QR pattern found in 18 patients, an Rs in 1 patient, an RS in 1 patient, an rs in 2 patients, an rsR′ in 1 patient, and an rsr′ in 1 patient. Assessment of the left precordial leads after ablation showed that in only 9 patients, the previous ECG pattern changed with the development of a small q wave, while the other patients showed the same pre-ablation QRS complex. Figure 3.2 shows examples when comparing the QRS pre- and postablation.

Correlation between ECG findings and Mahaim fiber location

The rS morphology in lead III was not seen in the 3 patients with an anteriorly located Mahaim or in the 2 patients with a posterior Mahaim. The distribution of the atrial end of the Mahaim fiber in the 20 patients with an rS pattern in lead III during sinus rhythm around the tricuspid annulus is depicted in Fig. 3.5. It is of interest that the atrial end of the Mahaim fiber with an rS pattern in lead III can be found over a large area around the tricuspid annulus, from the anterolateral to the posterolateral and midseptal region.

The presence of an rS pattern in lead III during sinus rhythm in 200 matched controls

We did a survey in 200 matched controls (56% female patients with a mean age of 23 ± 12 yr) without heart disease and without a history of palpitations. Twelve out of these 200 (6%) showed an rS pattern in lead III during sinus rhythm (Table 3.3). However, all of them had a q wave in lead I (qR or qRs patterns)

Discussion

When accessory AV pathways have conduction times approaching that of the normal AV conduction system, little or no preexcitation may be present during sinus rhythm. The reported incidence of minimal preexcitation in the 12-lead ECG during sinus rhythm in patients with decrementally conducting accessory

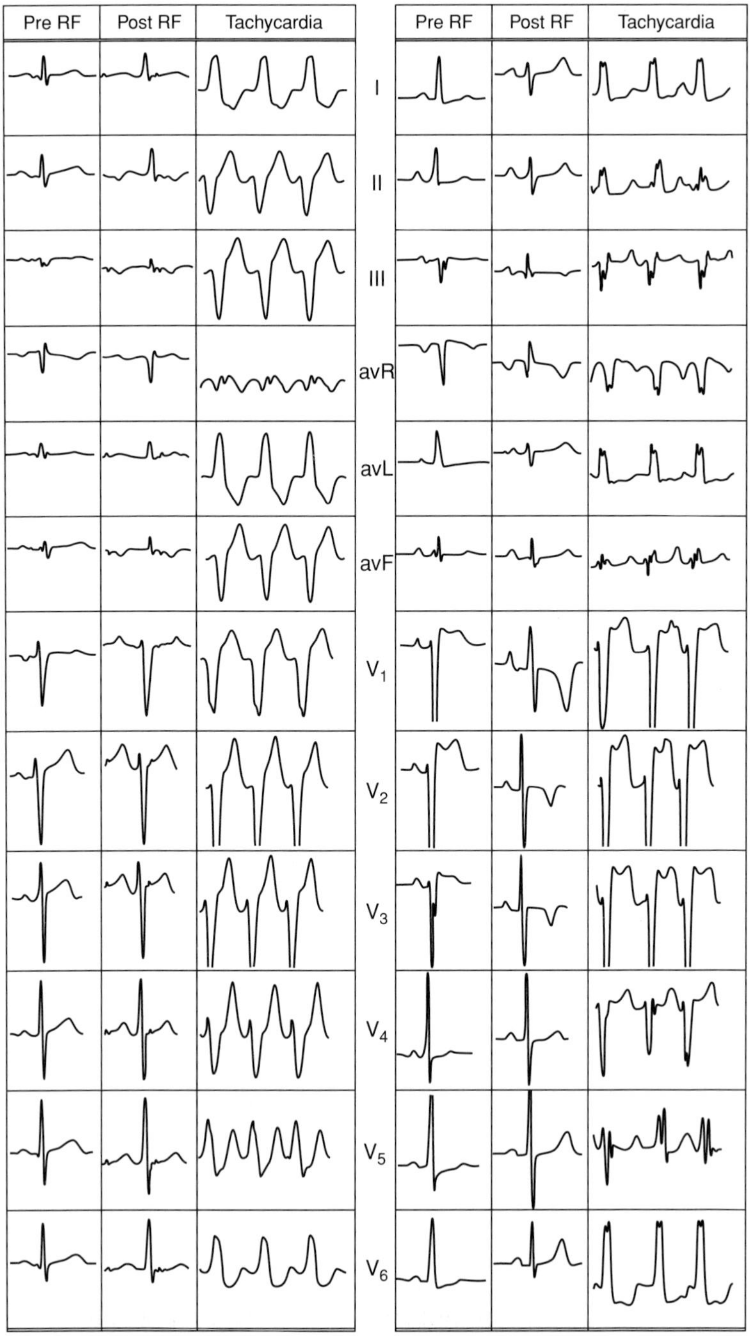

Figure 3.3 Two patients with an atriofascicular pathway displaying the rS pattern in lead III. Pre/post, pre- or post-RF catheter ablation.

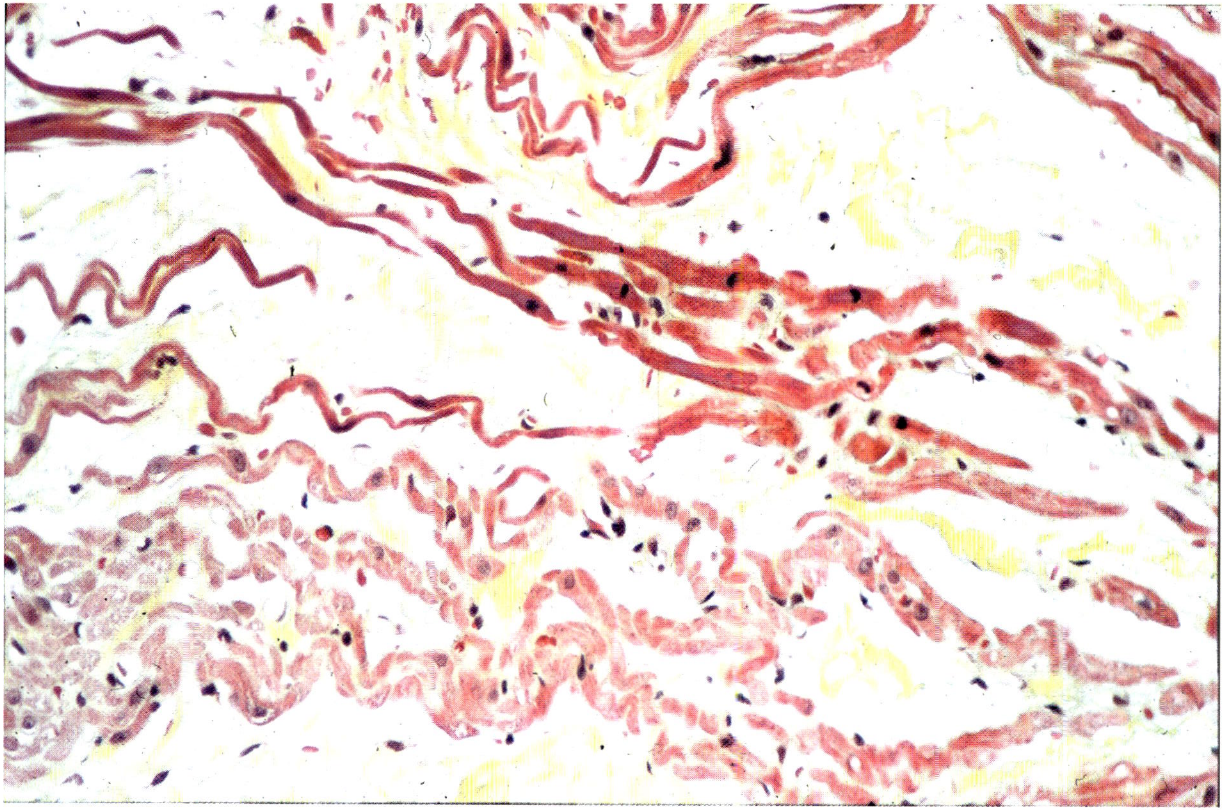

Plate 1 This photomicrograph of an accessory AV node (HE stain) shows myofibrils of normal size and aspect in the lower segment. In the upper segment the myofibrils are slender and isolated in small bundles by connective tissue, suggesting the presence of a highly complex system network. Courtesy of Drs Colette and Gerard Guiraudon.

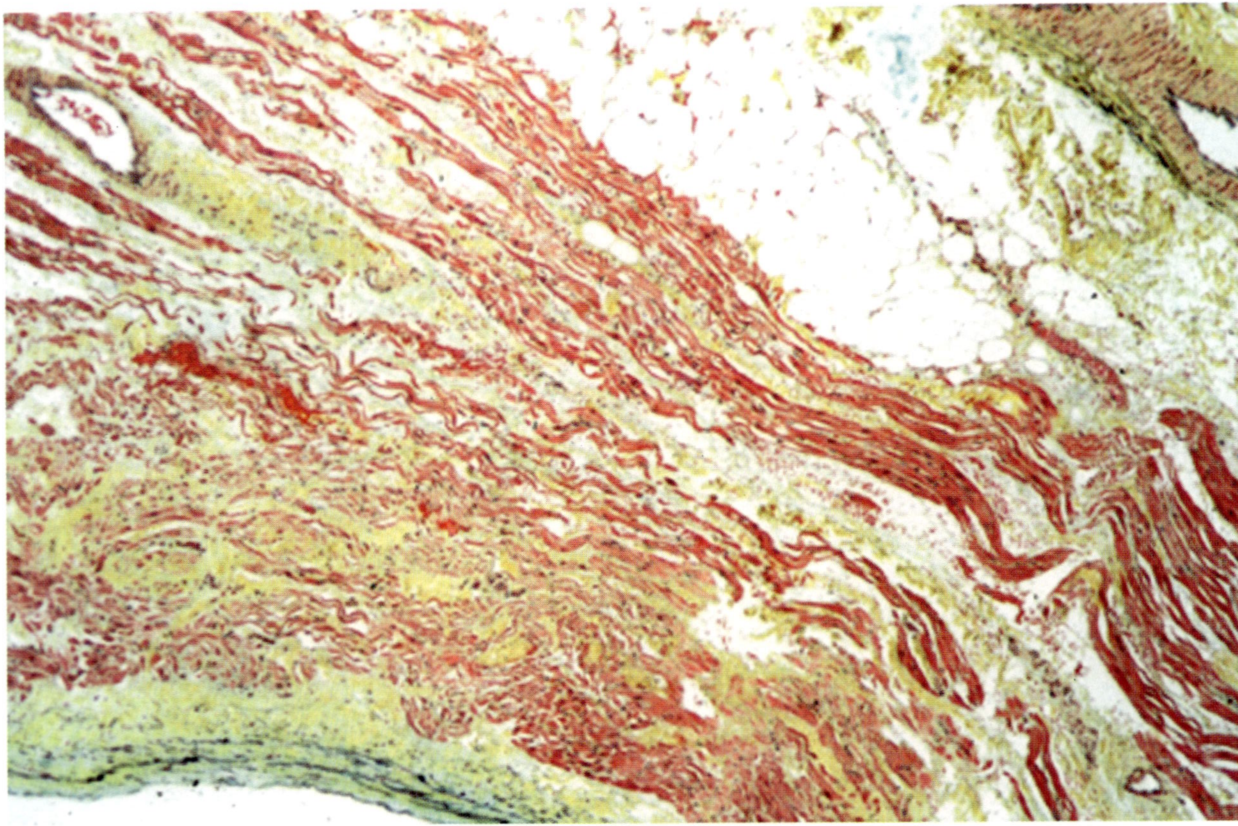

Plate 2 A morphological pattern similar to that in Fig. 2.1 is shown for another patient. There is normal atrial myocardium in the left lower part and slender myofibrils in the right upper part organized in bundles by septa of fatty or connective tissue. Courtesy of Drs Colette and Gerard Guiraudon.

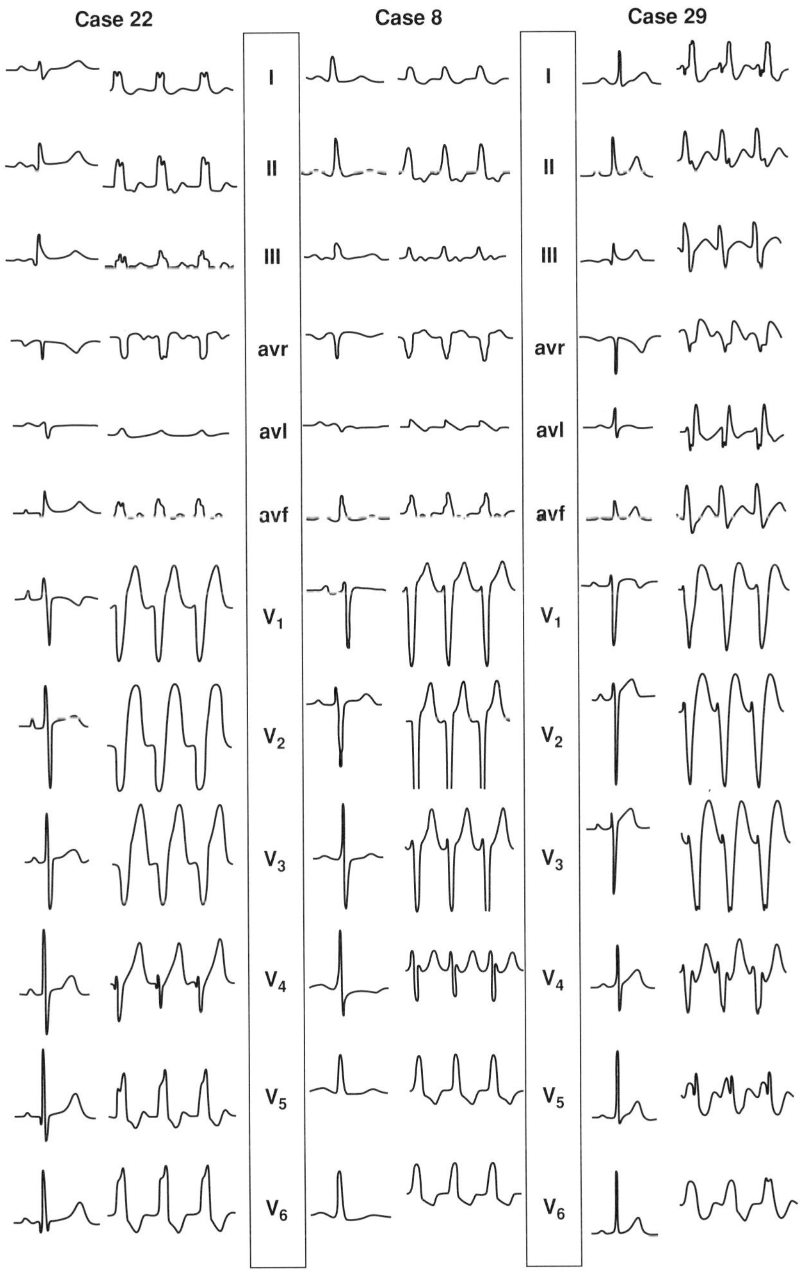

Figure 3.4 Cases 22, 8, and 29: these patients had an anterior Mahaim fiber and an intermediate QRS axis (60°, 50°, and 50°, respectively) during sinus rhythm and antidromic tachycardia. There is a minimal preexcitation but without the rS pattern in lead III.

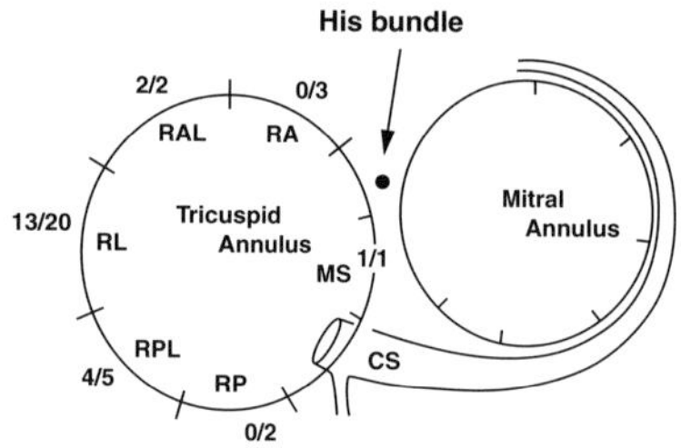

Figure 3.5 Proportion of patients with an rS pattern in lead III during sinus rhythm in relation to the location of the atrial end of the Mahaim fiber along the tricuspid annulus. Abbreviations: MS, midseptal; CS, coronary sinus; RA, right anterior; RAL, right anterolateral; RL, right lateral; RP, right posterior; RPL, right posterolateral.

pathways is low. Bardy *et al.* [16] and Klein *et al.* [18] did not find it in any of their patients. McClelland *et al.* [13] reported that only one of his 26 patients displayed preexcitation on the 12-lead ECG. When we realized the prevalence of the rS pattern in lead III in our patients, we examined previous reports dealing with decrementally conducting bypass tracts. We did find the rS pattern in lead III in many ECGs considered as normal in cardiology journals [17, 12–23] and textbooks [24–25]. This suggests that the reported low figures of abnormal ECGs in patients with Mahaim bypass tracts is an underestimation. Some authors did acknowledge the presence of minimal preexcitation in 25% to 50% of the patients [14, 18]. We found an incidence of 72% of minimal preexcitation, mainly in the presence of an rS pattern in lead III (60%). It should be stressed that in these patients there is no classic delta wave. It is of interest that the rS pattern was found in patients with decremental accessory pathways having their atrial end over a very large area around the tricuspid annulus, from anterolateral to posterolateral, and also in the only patient with a midseptal location (Fig. 3.5). This supports a ventricular insertion in a small anterolateral area in the right ventricle in or close to the exit of the right bundle branch and also explains (when ventricular activation starts at this site) the absence of a q wave in lead I.

To validate the rS and rsR′ as abnormal patterns in lead III due to preexcitation of a small region of the right ventricle, it was critical to show a positive relationship between those patterns in lead III during sinus rhythm and left-axis deviation during tachycardia with anterograde conduction over the Mahaim

Table 3.3 Lead III pattern in 200 young individuals with palpitations.

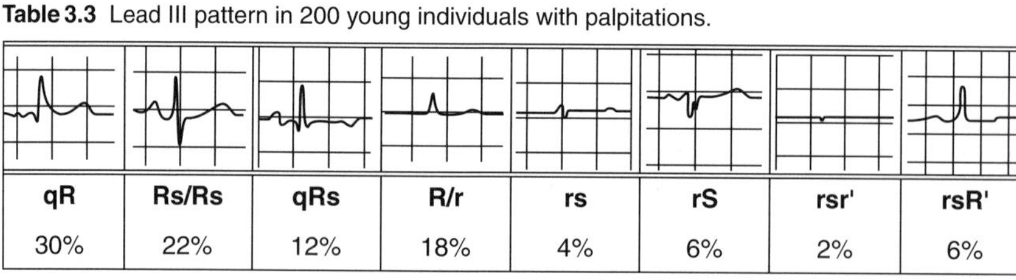

qR	Rs/Rs	qRs	R/r	rs	rS	rsr'	rsR'
30%	22%	12%	18%	4%	6%	2%	6%

fiber (Fig. 3.3). All 20 patients with an rS in lead III had left-axis deviation ($\leq 0°$) during tachycardia. Another important step in validation is to show a clear change in QRS complex configuration after ablation of the decremental accessory pathway. Figure 3.2 depicts most of the patterns of QRS that emerged after successful ablation of the Mahaim fiber.

The fact that 9 patients did not show an rS pattern in lead III during sinus rhythm but an LBBB-like QRS with left-axis deviation during tachycardia can be explained by impulse conduction over the Mahaim fiber during sinus rhythm slower than impulse conduction over the normal AV conduction system. We, like other authors [26], found day to-day variability in the expression of minimal preexcitation. This is different from "intermittent" preexcitation, which may occur in rapidly conducting APs with long anterograde refractory periods. Our patients with variable expression of preexcitation did not have long refractory periods of their accessory pathway. There is one case report of sudden death in a patient with similar findings [27]. Conduction over Mahaim fibers can be so slow that no ventricular preexcitation occurs even during atrial pacing. Still, these so-called latent Mahaim fibers are capable of being involved in antidromic tachycardias [28].

Are all Mahaim fibers inserting close to or in the right bundle branch?

Some Mahaim fibers are probably not inserting in that region. Our 3 patients with anterior Mahaim did not show an rS in lead III nor left-axis deviation during tachycardia, suggesting that in those fibers, the ventricular insertion is not in the vicinity of the right bundle branch [6] (Fig. 3.4).

Septal q waves

In our population lead I was more sensitive for minimal preexcitation than lead V_6. In patients with atriofascicular pathways inserting close to the apex, ventricular activation proceeds from an apical toward a basal direction, resulting in a q wave in lead V_6. Minimal preexcitation due to left-sided accessory pathways can be better appreciated in lead V_6, which has been shown to be more sensitive than leads I and avL [29].

"rS" as a normal pattern in lead III

It has been shown [30] that an rS pattern in lead III can be found in normal individuals. This may occur during posterior displacement of the apex leading to S waves in leads I, II, and III (*S1S2S3* pattern) [31] and in counterclockwise rotation of the heart resulting in a qR in lead I and an rS in lead III. However, in those situations a normal q wave in lead I is likely to be present. In our survey on 200 ECGs from young individuals with palpitations, we found the rS pattern in lead III in 6% but always associated with a q wave in lead I. No individual showed an rS pattern in lead III combined with the absence of a q wave in lead I, a pattern that seems specific for patients with a Mahaim fiber.

Limitation of the study specificity of the rS pattern in the general population

The finding of an rS pattern in lead III in 60% of the patients with Mahaim fibers is significantly higher than its occurrence in young persons with palpitations ($p < 0.0001$).

Mahaim fibers comprise approximately 3% of the overt accessory pathways [32]. Based on the prevalence of accessory pathways in the general population [33] (0.2%), the prevalence of Mahaim fibers would be 0.5–1:10 000. The specificity of an rS pattern in lead III associated with the absence of a septal q wave will be close to 90% (if we assume one false positive in 1000 individuals), albeit the sensitivity decreases to 45%.

Conclusion

In young patients suffering from tachycardias the finding of a narrow QRS with an rS pattern in lead III during sinus rhythm should raise the suspicion of the presence of a Mahaim fiber, especially in those showing absence of a q wave in lead I.

The ECG during tachycardia: Old criteria revisited

Twenty years ago Bardy *et al.* [16] reported six ECG features showing a high efficacy in identifying antidromic tachycardia due to nodofascicular (NF) accessory pathways. In that study all 22 ECGs with ventricular tachycardia (VT) were correctly identified and only 1 of 18 ECGs with antidromic tachycardia was not diagnosed as a Mahaim tachycardia. Those criteria – (i) a QRS axis between 0° and −75°, (ii) a QRS duration of 0.15 seconds or less, (iii) an R wave in limb lead I, (iv) an rS in precordial lead V_1, (v) a transition in the precordial leads from a predominantly positive QRS complex greater than V_4, and (vi) a tachycardia cycle length between 220 and 450 milliseconds – became the gold standard in identifying preexcited tachycardia due to anterograde conduction over a decrementally conducting accessory pathway. In the following decades our understanding about the anatomic course as well as the site of the proximal and distal insertion of such pathways has evolved [4, 5, 11, 13, 18, 22, 34–37]. Those pathways originally described as NF fibers would probably be reclassified today as atriofascicular pathways or decrementally conducting accessory AV pathways. The aim of our study was to evaluate the sensitivity, specificity, and positive and negative predictive value of the criteria from the study of Bardy *et al.* to identify patients with a tachycardia using a right-sided atriofascicular or decrementally conducting accessory AV pathway with emphasis on the differential diagnosis with LBBB-shaped supraventricular tachycardia (SVT).

Definitions of terms

Short decremental AV pathways

During preexcited tachycardia there was a long VH interval with early ventricular activation at the tricuspid annulus and late activation of the RV apex.

Long decremental right superior ("anterior") AV pathways

During preexcited tachycardia there was late activation of the RV apex and at the tricuspid annulus, and the 12-lead ECG did not have left-axis deviation (QRS frontal plane axis between $+30^\circ$ and $+60^\circ$).

Atrial insertion was located by the finding of the Mahaim ("M") potential at the right superior area at the tricuspid annulus.

Accessory pathway location nomenclature was presented in accordance with a previous expert consensus statement [38].

We classified these patients with Mahaim fibers into two groups: group I with 32 patients with right-sided atriofascicular pathways (Fig. 3.6) and group II with 5 patients with a short decrementally conducting right-sided AV pathway characterized by a distal insertion close to the tricuspid annulus (Fig. 3.7) plus 3 patients with long right superior decrementally conducting AV pathways (Fig. 3.8). As a control group we examined 35 patients with SVT and aberrant conduction with an LBBB-shaped QRS (group III). All tracings were reviewed by the authors and two cardiologists to assess interobserver variability.

The 40 consecutive patients with decrementally conducting accessory pathways (Tables 3.4 and 3.5) came from four institutions. There were 23 female patients and 17 male patients, with a mean age of 25 ± 13 (range 8–80) years. Thirty-two patients underwent RF catheter ablation at the atrial side of the tricuspid annulus where a discrete accessory pathway ("M") potential was

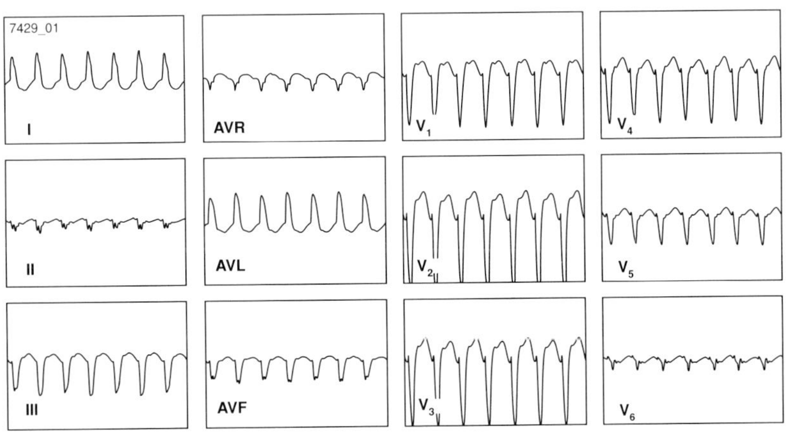

Figure 3.6 A 12-lead ECG obtained during antidromic tachycardia in a patient with an anterior (right lateral) atriofascicular pathway (QRS = 0.12 s).

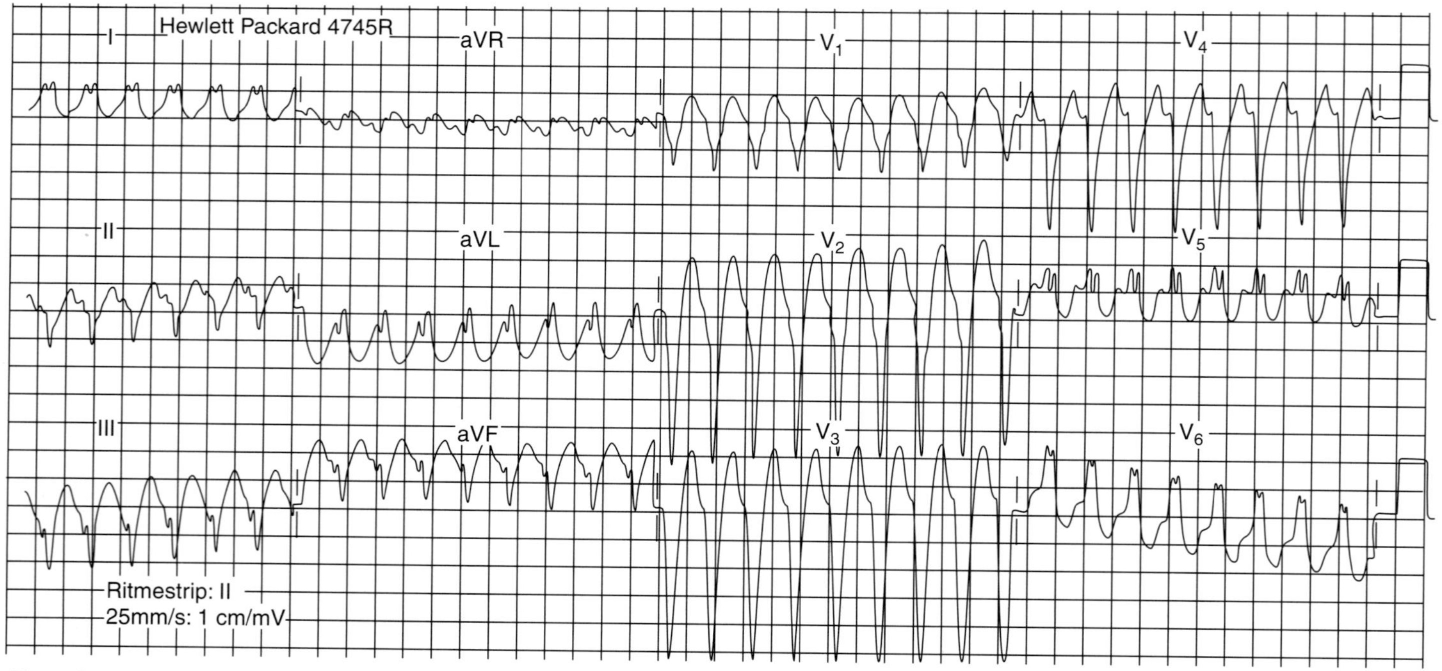

Figure 3.7 A 12-lead ECG during antidromic tachycardia in a patient with a short decrementally AV accessory pathway (QRS = 0.17 s).

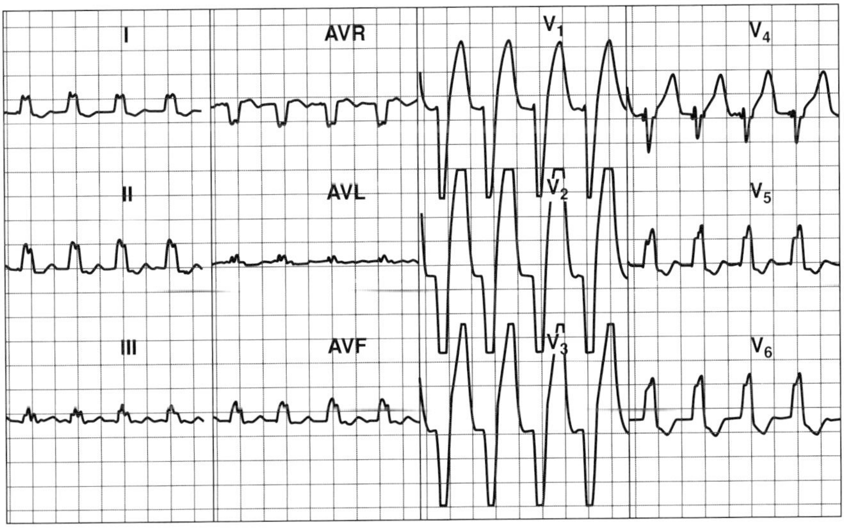

Figure 3.8 A 12-lead ECG during antidromic tachycardia in a patient with a long superior (right anterior) decrementally accessory AV pathway (QRS = 0.16 s).

recorded, while in five patients (patients 1, 2, 4, 7, and 8, Table 3.4, AV Mahaim section) catheter ablation was carried out at the ventricular insertion guided by the pace-mapping technique. In 2 patients the pathway was surgically interrupted. In all patients the accessory pathway was successfully ablated.

The control group consisted of 35 patients (60% female) with an LBBB-shaped SVT and a mean age of 40 ± 20 years (Table 3.4).

Results

ECG during preexcited tachycardia in patients with an atriofascicular pathway (group I)

The index arrhythmia in the 32 patients with atriofascicular pathways was antidromic tachycardia with anterograde conduction over the atriofascicular pathway in 25 patients. There was an incessant nonsustained spontaneous automatic tachycardia arising in the atriofascicular pathway in 2 patients. A preexcited tachycardia due to AVNRT with bystander anterograde atriofascicular conduction was present in one patient, preexcited atrial fibrillation in one patient, and antidromic tachycardia with anterograde conduction over the atriofascicular pathway and retrograde conduction with fusion between the AV node and a rapidly conducting accessory pathway (two right inferior paraseptal and one anterior) in 3 patients. These 3 patients with multiple accessory pathways also had an additional inducible orthodromic AV reentrant tachycardia. Mean cycle length of the preexcited tachycardia was 332 ± 39 milliseconds (range 220 to 420). Mean QRS width was 127 ± 8 milliseconds (range 120–150).

Table 3.4 Clinical data of patients with Mahaim fibers.

Case	*Age*	*Gender*	*Right sided AFP site*	*C. Diagnosis*	*AP site*	*Ebstein*	*Therapy*
1	32	F	AI	AVNRT			RF_p
2	19	F	AI			Yes	RF_p
3	21	F	AI			Yes	RF_p
4	13	M	AI	WPW	IPS	Yes	RF_p
5	52	M	AI				RF_p
6	21	M	AI				RF_p
7	8	F	SA				RF_p
8	30	M	AI				RF_p
9	27	F	A				RF_p
10	19	F	A				RF_p
11	12	F	Septal				RF_p
12	39	F	A				RF_p
13	15	M	SA				RF_p
14	17	M	A	WPW/CBT	IPS/A	Yes	RF_p
15	23	F	A	AVNRT			RF_p
16	80	M	AI	WPW	IPS		RF_p
17	25	F	AI				RF_p
18	35	M	A				RF_p
19	42	F	A				RF_p
20	23	F	A				RF_p
21	23	F	A				RF_p
22	45	F	A				RF_p
23	23	M	A				S
24	11	M	A			Yes	RF-dis
25	26	M	A	CBT	P	Yes	RF-dis
26	26	F	A	AVNRT			RF-dis
27	31	F	A				RF-dis
28	22	F	A				RF_p
29	17	M	I				RF_p
30	18	F	A				RF_p
31	31	F	A				S
32	8	M	A				RF_p
Mean $\pm$ SD $= 26 \pm 14$							
			AVP Site				
1	31	M	A				RF_p
2	12	F	A	WPW	A	Yes	RF_p
3	15	M	S				RF_p
4	17	F	A				RF_p
5	25	M	S				RF-dis
6	19	F	S				RF_p
7	50	F	AI				RF_p
8	25	M	A				RF_p
Mean $\pm$ SD $= 24 \pm 10$							

A, anterior*; AFP site, atriofascicular pathway–right atrial insertion; AI, anteroinferior; AVP, AV Mahaim fiber; C, concomitant; CBT, concealed bypass tract; I, inferior; IPS, inferoparaseptal; P, posterior; S, superior; SA, superoanterior.

Therapy: RFp, catheter ablation targeting the atrial insertion guided by the proximal AP (M) potential; RFd, catheter ablation at the distal insertion of the Mahaim fiber; S, surgical endocardial ablation.

Table 3.5 Electrocardiographic characteristics of the pre-excited tachycardia.

AF Mahaim	Cycle length 220–450 ms	QRS (≤150 ms)	QRS axis (degrees)	Lead I configration	Lead V_1 configration	Precordial QRS transition	Preexcited tachycardia (anterograde, retrograde pathways)	False–
1	280	130	−20	R	LBBB(rS)	V_5	AF, His	
2	240	140	−60	R	LBBB(rS)	V_6	AF, His	
3	300	130	−60	R	LBBB(rS)	V_6	AF, His	
4	320	150	−45	R	LBBB(rS)	V_5	AF, PS AP + His	
5	330	130	−45	R	LBBB(rS)	$>V_6$	preexcited (AF) Afib	
6	310	120	−30	**qR**	LBBB(rS)	V_6	AF, His	×
7	380	120	0	R	LBBB(rS)	V_5	Mahaim automaticity	
8	380	150	−60	R	LBBB(rS)	V_5	AF, His	
9	390	130	−30	R	LBBB(rS)	V_6	AF, His	
10	320	130	−30	R	LBBB(rS)	V_6	AF, His	
11	420	120	−60	R	LBBB(rS)	V_5	Mahaim automaticity	
12	320	140	−45	R	LBBB(rS)	$>V_6$	AF, His	
13	330	140	0	R	LBBB(rS)	V_5	AF, His	
14	330	130	0	R	LBBB(rS)	V_5	AF, RL cAP + His	
15	320	120	−15	R	LBBB(rS)	V_5	AVNRT + bystander AF	
16	310	120	0	R	LBBB(rS)	V_5	AF, PS AP + His	
17	300	130	−45	R	LBBB(rS)	V_6	AF, His	

Continued p. 32

Table 3.5 (*Continued*)

AF Mahaim	*Cycle length 220–450 ms*	*QRS (≤150 ms)*	*QRS axis (degrees)*	*Lead I configration*	*Lead V_1 configration*	*Precordial QRS transition*	*Preexcited tachycardia (anterograde, retrograde pathways)*	*False–*
18	340	120	−60	R	LBBB(rS)	**V_4**	AF, His	×
19	340	120	−15	R	LBBB(rS)	V_6	AF, His	
20	350	130	−30	R	LBBB(rS)	$> V_6$	AF, His	
21	300	120	−30	R	LBBB(rS)	V_5	AF, His	
22	380	120	−30	R	LBBB(rS)	V_6	AF, His	
23	320	120	−60	R	LBBB(rS)	V_5	AF, His	
24	350	120	0	R	LBBB(rS)	V_5	AF, His	
25	300	120	−75	R	LBBB(rS)	V_5	AF, LL cAP + His	
26	400	120	−60	R	**LBBB(QS)**	$> V_6$	AF, His	×
27	300	120	−60	R	LBBB(rS)	V_6	AF, His	
28	400	130	−30	R	LBBB(rS)	V_5	AF, His	
29	280	130	−15	R	LBBB(rS)	V_5	AF, His	
30	340	130	0	R	LBBB(rS)	V_5	AF, His	
31	340	130	**20**	R	LBBB(rS)	V_5	AF, His	×
32	310	130	−30	R	LBBB(rS)	V_5	AF, His	
Mean ± SD	332 ± 39	127 ± 8	(−31) ± 24					4/32 (12.5 %)

1	400	160	−5	R	LBBB(rS)	V_5	AV, His	×
2	240	**200**	−15	R	LBBB(rS)	V_6	AV, RL WPW + His	×
3	420	**160**	**45**	R	LBBB(rS)	V_5	AV, His	×
4	280	**180**	−75	R	**LBBB(QS)**	V_6	AV, His	×
5	320	**160**	**30**	**rsR'**	LBBB(rS)	V_5	AV, His	×
6	310	140	**50**	R	LBBB(rS)	V_5	AV, His	×
7	320	**160**	−75	R	**LBBB(QS)**	V_6	AV, His	×
8	310	**160**	−30	R	LBBB(rS)	V_5	AVNRT + bystander AV	×
								8/8 (100 %)
Mean ± SD	325 ± 59	165 ± 17	(−9) ± 49					
P value	P = ns	$P < 0.0001$	$P = 0.07$					

A, anterior; AF, atriofascicular; AV, decrementally conducting AV accessory pathway; CAP, concealed accessory pathway; Mahaim automaticity, automaticity arising in the decremental pathway; RIPS, right inferoparaseptal; LBBB, left bundle branch block-like pattern; P, posterior.

No patient with an atriofascicular pathway had a QRS greater than 150 milliseconds. Mean QRS axis was -31 ± 24 (range 20 to -75) degrees, but only one patient with an atriofascicular pathway showed a positive frontal plane axis during preexcited tachycardia. All patients with atriofascicular pathways showed an R wave in lead I, except patient 6 (qR). Thirty-one patients showed an rS pattern in lead V_1 (patient 26 had a QS pattern). The QRS transition in the precordial leads (R/S >1) occurred after V_4 in all but patient 18. Sensitivity of all six criteria in identifying an atriofascicular pathway was 87.5% in these 32 patients. There were four false negatives.

ECG during preexcited tachycardia in patients with an AV accessory pathway with decremental conduction (group II)

The index arrhythmia in 7 of 8 patients was an antidromic tachycardia using the Mahaim fiber as the anterograde limb of the circuit. In 6 patients the AV node–His bundle–right bundle branch system was used as the retrograde limb, while in patient 2, ventriculoatrial (VA) conduction occurred over the AV node and a right lateral rapidly conducting accessory pathway. One patient had AVNRT with bystander anterograde conduction over a short AV Mahaim fiber (patient 8). The mean tachycardia cycle length was 325 ± 59 milliseconds (range 240–420) and within the previously described range. The mean QRS complex width (165 ± 17 ms) was larger than the width of the QRS in patients with atriofascicular pathways ($p < 0.0001$). Five of the seven patients had a QRS complex width above the 150-milliseconds limit. The mean frontal plane axis (-9 ± 49) in these patients was not significantly different ($p = 0.07$) from that of the patients with an atriofascicular pathway in spite of a trend toward a less-marked left-axis deviation. Six patients showed an R wave in lead I, and 6 patients showed an rS pattern in lead V_1. No patient with an AV Mahaim would be diagnosed using the criteria from the study by Bardy *et al.* Those exclusions were based on the presence of three different criteria in 1 patient, two criteria in 3 patients, and only one criterion in 4 patients. No exclusions occurred by the criterion "cycle length."

Control group (group III)

The control group, consisting of patients with SVT and LBBB aberrant conduction, had a similar gender distribution but with a higher mean age (40 ± 20 yr, $p < 0.001$). The tachycardia mechanisms were A-V reentry with V-A conduction over a rapidly conducting accessory pathway in 19 patients (14 left free-wall), AVNRT in 11 patients (1 slow-slow and 10 slow-fast), and atrial reentry in five patients (Table 3.6). Mean tachycardia cycle length of 331 ± 60 milliseconds was similar to the patients from groups I and II ($p =$ ns). The mean QRS complex width (153 ± 23 ms) was also larger than the width of the QRS in patients with atriofascicular pathways ($p < 0.0001$) but not different from the group II patients (165 ± 17 ms, $p =$ ns). The patients with atrial reentry showed the widest QRS width (188 ± 18 ms). The mean frontal plane axis $+10^\circ \pm 49^\circ$) in these patients was also significantly different ($p < 0.0001$) from the axis in

Table 3.6 Electrocardiographic characteristics of the LBBB-shaped SVT.

Case	Cycle length 220–450 ms	QRS ms	QRS axis (0 to 75 degrees)	Lead I R	Lead V_1 rS	Precordial QRS transition	Tachycardia circuit	Diagnosis	False +
1	340	130	–60	Yes	Yes	V_5	AVRT	P CBT	×
2	320	140	**50**	Yes	Yes	$\mathbf{V_4}$	AVRT	P CBT	
3	240	**180**	**60**	Yes	**No**	$\mathbf{V_4}$	AVRT	RIPS WPW	
4	240	**160**	–10	Yes	**No**	V_5	slow-fast	AVNRT	
5	260	140	–20	Yes	Yes	V_5	slow-fast	AVNRT	×
6	430	**200**	**90**	**No(RS)**	**No**	V_5	focal RAT/preexistent LBBB	AT	
7	480	**180**	**50**	Yes	Yes	$\mathbf{V_4}$	atrial flutter/preexistent LBBB	Atrial flutter	
8	360	**170**	–45	Yes	Yes	V_6	slow-fast	AVNRT	
9	360	140	0	Yes	**No**	V_5	AVRT	P CBT	
10	340	140	–60	Yes	**No**	V_5	AVRT	P CBT	
11	280	**200**	0	Yes	**No**	$\mathbf{V_3}$	slow-fast	AVNRT	
12	260	**160**	**60**	Yes	**No**	V_5	AVRT	P CBT	
13	310	140	**75**	**No(r)**	Yes	V_6	AVRT	A WPW	
14	300	140	**75**	**No(qr)**	Yes	V_6	slow-fast	AVNRT	
15	480	**160**	**45**	**No(rS)**	Yes	V_5	focal RAT/preexistent LBBB	AT	
16	300	**200**	**15**	Yes	**No**	V_6	focal RAT	AT	
17	350	**170**	–15	Yes	Yes	$\mathbf{V_4}$	slow-fast	AVNRT	
18	250	150	0	Yes	**No**	V_5	slow-fast	AVNRT	
19	310	**180**	**60**	**No(Rs)**	**No**	$\mathbf{V_4}$	AVRT	LIPS CBT	

Continued p. 36

Table 3.6 (*Continued*)

Case	*Cycle length 220–450 ms*	*QRS ms*	*QRS axis (0 to 75 degrees)*	*Lead I R*	*Lead V_1 rS*	*Precordial QRS transition*	*Tachycardia circuit*	*Diagnosis*	*False +*
20	450	**200**	**60**	Yes	Yes	V_5	focal RAT/preexistent LBBB	AT	
21	320	**180**	−60	Yes	**No**	V_5	AVRT	PI CBT	
22	400	140	−45	Yes	Yes	$\mathbf{V_4}$	AVRT	P WPW	
23	320	140	**60**	Yes	Yes	$\mathbf{V_4}$	AVRT	P WPW	
24	320	140	**−90**	**No(RS)**	Yes	$\mathbf{V_4}$	slow-fast	AVNRT	
25	290	**160**	−60	**No(qR)**	**No**	V_6	slow-fast	AVNRT	
26	320	140	**60**	Yes	Yes	V_5	AVRT	P CBT	
27	320	120	**45**	Yes	Yes	$\mathbf{V_4}$	slow-fast	AVNRT	
28	320	130	0	Yes	Yes	V_6	AVRT	P WPW	×
29	290	140	−30	Yes	**No**	V_5	slow-slow	AVNRT	
30	320	130	**60**	Yes	Yes	$\mathbf{V_4}$	AVRT	P CBT	
31	310	130	−30	Yes	Yes	V_5	AVRT	P CBT	×
32	310	140	**30**	Yes	Yes	V_5	AVRT	P WPW	
33	400	140	−30	Yes	Yes	V_6	AVRT	P WPW	×
34	320	130	**30**	Yes	Yes	V_5	AVRT	P CBT	
35	380	130	−30	Yes	Yes	$> V_6$	AVRT	SPS CBT	×
Mean ± SD	331 ± 60	153 ± 23	10 ± 49						6/35 pts(17.4 %)

A, anterior; AP, accessory pathway; AVNP, AV node pathway; CBT, concealed bypass tract; P, posterior; PI, posteroinferior; RAT, right atrial tachycardia; RIPS, right inferoparaseptal; SPS, superoparaseptal; WPW, Wolff-Parkinson-White.

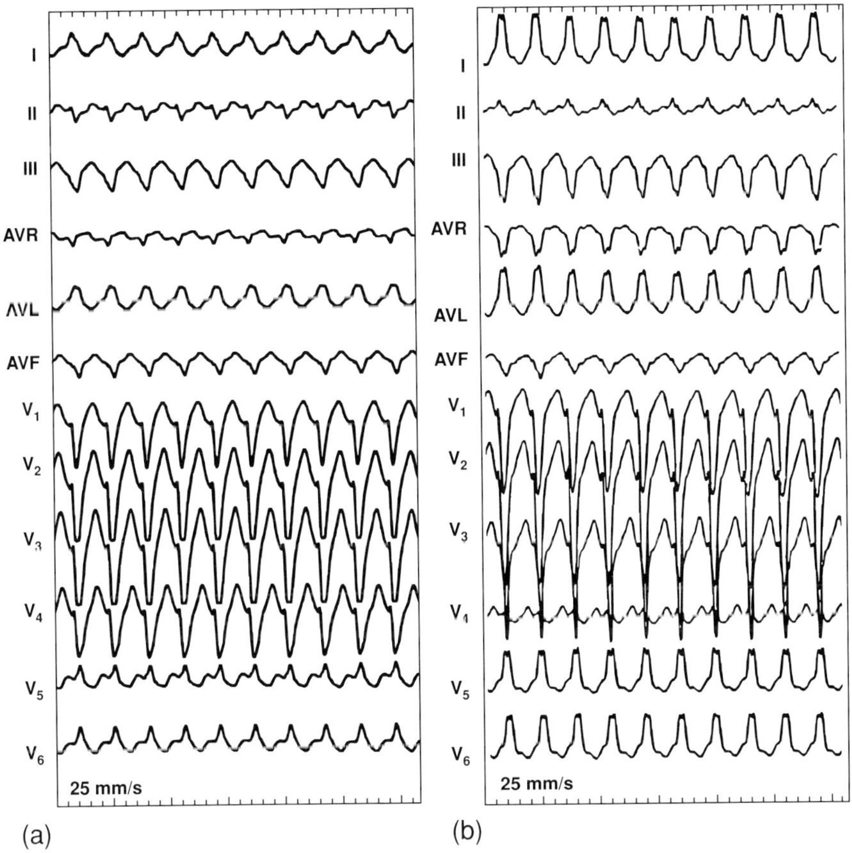

Figure 3.9 (a) An LBBB-shaped tachycardia due to AV reentry in a patient with a concealed left free-wall accessory pathway. (b) Antidromic tachycardia with anterograde conduction over an atriofascicular pathway. Applying the criteria from the study of Bardy *et al.*, both tachyarrhythmias would be classified as a group I tachycardia (see text).

patients with an atriofascicular pathway but not significantly different from group II patients. Six patients (17%) would be erroneously (false positives) diagnosed as having a Mahaim tachycardia. The most frequent finding associated with a false positive was the presence of an accessory pathway. Five of the 19 patients with AV orthodromic tachycardia with aberrant LBBB (26%) would be misclassified (Fig. 3.9). One of 11 patients (9%) with AVNRT and aberrant LBBB would be classified as a tachycardia using an atriofascicular pathway. No patient with an atrial tachycardia due to atrial reentry was misclassified. Correct identification of aberrant SVT was done by five criteria in 1 patient, four in 2 patients, three in 7 patients, two in 10 patients, and only one criterion in 9 patients.

Interobserver variability

Comparative analysis of the 74 12-lead ECGs with LBBB-shaped tachycardia by the four observers resulted in no disagreement.

Discussion

Ventricular activation during a QRS with LBBB configuration

Our understanding of ventricular activation during LBBB in humans is based on intraoperative epicardial studies [39], catheter-based endocardial mapping studies [40], and an endocardial mapping study by using a noncontact catheter technique [41]. These studies showed that in most patients with LBBB, activation started in the anterior RV wall. The delayed left septal activation (the septum is activated from right to left and usually in an anteroposterior direction) causes disappearance of the q wave in leads I and aVL and in the left precordial leads and also of the r wave in V_1 in up to 50% of the patients. The activation of the anterior region of the RV can explain the inscription of a small and narrow r wave in lead V_1 in the other half. In 97% of the group I patients with an atriofascicular pathway the presence of an r wave in lead V_1 is consistent with preexcitation of the anterior region of the RV, close to the area where the right bundle branch connects to the RV myocardium. On the other hand, as expected, 37% of our patients with an LBBB-shaped SVT show a QS pattern in lead V_1. In spite of a mean axis of -31° the wide range in frontal QRS axis from 0 to -75° can be explained by the variable site of early activation of the right ventricle and left ventricular septal activation in the presence of LBBB: anteroseptal, posteroseptal (close to the posterior fascicle), or midseptal [41].

LBBB tachycardia in patients with decrementally conducting accessory AV pathways

The causes of failure to correctly identify these patients are twofold:

1 the absence of left-axis deviation in the three patients with a long superior AV Mahaim, whose distal insertion is not in the vicinity of the distal right bundle branch;

2 a wider QRS found in patients with a short decremental AV fiber, leading to a ventricular preexcitation pattern like that of a rapidly conducting right-sided bypass tract

Six of the group II 8 patients had a QRS width of more than 150 milliseconds.

LBBB-shaped SVT

The higher age of the control group can be explained by the inclusion of patients with atrial reentry and AVNRT whose incidence peaks after the fourth decade. Our finding that 5 of the 6 false positives in the control group were caused by AV reentrant tachycardia using an accessory pathway highlights the importance of the tachycardia mechanism. As long as 26% of the LBBB SVT due to an accessory pathway falls within the false positive range, a higher proportion of orthodromic tachycardia in the control group can decrease the negative predictive value of the aforementioned criteria, and vice versa: the more patients with SVT and preexistent LBBB are included, the higher the positive predictive value, because this group of patients has a mean larger QRS width (188 ± 18 milliseconds).

Comparison of our data with the study of Bardy *et al.*

The small differences between our data and the results reported by the group from Duke University, sensitivity (87.5% vs. 92%, $p = 0.9$) and negative predictive values (82.5% vs. 91%, $p = 0.5$) of the six electrocardiographic criteria did not reach statistical significance. The criterion cycle length was not helpful in our study as in Bardy's series.

All electrocardiographic criteria are simple, easy to assess, with no interobserver variability, and only the QRS transition in the precordial leads can be influenced by a malpositioning of the electrodes, but that would have the least impact on the results: one more false negative each in groups I and III.

Conclusion

The previously reported criteria showed reliable efficacy in identifying patients with an atriofascicular pathway but are of no value in distinguishing a decrementally conducting AV pathway from an atriofascicular pathway. The tachycardia cycle length was not helpful in making the correct diagnosis.

Electrophysiological aspects of atriofascicular pathways

Electrophysiological findings common to all decrementally conducting accessory pathways

During atrial pacing there is progressive AV and AH interval prolongation coupled with a decreasing HV interval resulting in a greater degree of ventricular preexcitation with an LBBB-like morphology in case of a right-sided pathway or an RBBB-like morphology with a left-sided Mahaim fiber [5, 8, 10]. In right-sided connections the His bundle deflection is inscribed after the right bundle potential during maximal preexcitation. At maximal ventricular preexcitation, there is a constant QRS-His relationship without further changes on shortening the atrial pacing cycle length.

Electrophysiological findings consistent with an atriofascicular pathway

During preexcited tachycardia there is a short V-RB interval because of early activation of the RV apex and late activation at the annulus. Proof of incorporation of the atriofascicular pathway as the anterograde limb of a circus movement tachycardia is the advancement of the following RV activation by delivering a late right atrial premature beat at the time of septal refractoriness (Fig. 3.10) [11]. However, it has been shown that inability to advance RV activation does not rule out the presence of an atriofascicular pathway nor its active role in the tachycardia circuit [12]. In those cases, definite proof can be provided by absence of ventricular preexcitation during atrial pacing and noninducibility of the tachycardia after successful ablation of the Mahaim fiber.

We have seen 5 patients with anterograde conduction over an atriofascicular pathway having a long VH preexcited tachycardia, either constant or

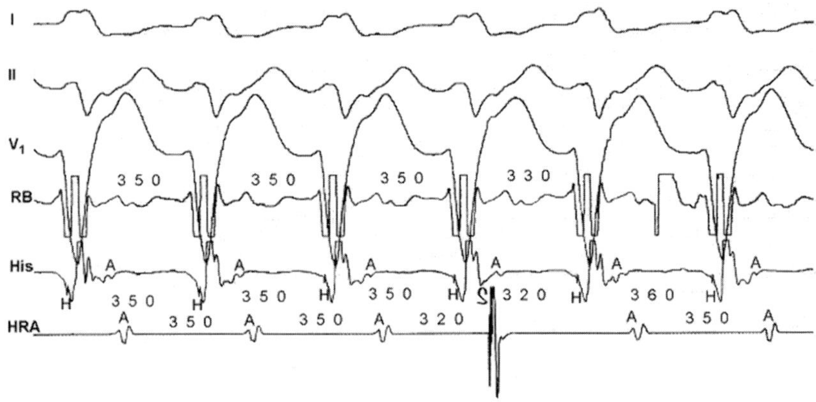

Figure 3.10 A late atrial premature beat (coupling interval of 320 ms) delivered at a time when His bundle refractoriness advanced the next ventricular and His bundle potential by 30 ms.

intermittent, because of persistent or transient RBBB, resulting in an increase of the tachycardia cycle length because of retrograde conduction over the left bundle branch. A similar phenomenon has been reported in patients with antidromic tachycardia using rapidly conducting accessory pathways [42]. In addition, in two of our patients with intermittent retrograde RBBB during antidromic tachycardia, we also found a frontal plane QRS axis shift to the left, causing a subtle change in the QRS morphology during preexcited long VH tachycardia (Figs. 3.11, 3.12, and 3.13) [43].

The atrial insertion can in most cases be located by finding an accessory pathway ("M") potential (Fig. 3.14). In some patients the "M" potential can be followed from the annulus to the distal end of the pathway [44]. Some authors have estimated its length as ranging from 2 to 5 cm [34, 36, 45]. Noncontact mapping during antidromic tachycardia in a patient with an atriofascicular pathway [36] showed conduction as far as at the RV apex, validating old data from intraoperative epicardial mapping [5]. However, it seems that some of the long Mahaim fibers do not connect into the distal RBB [18].

Electrophysiological findings consistent with a long decrementally AV accessory pathway

It is possible to differentiate an atriofascicular pathway, which connects to the distal Purkinje network of the right bundle branch, from a long and decrementally conducting AV pathway with a distal end connecting into the RV muscle at a variable distance from the exit of the right bundle branch. The following arguments favor a long decrementally conducting AV fiber:

1 The QRS duration and the V-His (and V-RB) interval during preexcited tachycardia. Our observations suggest that the distance between the myocardial insertion of the fiber and the right bundle branch is the key factor for those differences. A more pronounced slurring at the onset of the QRS during

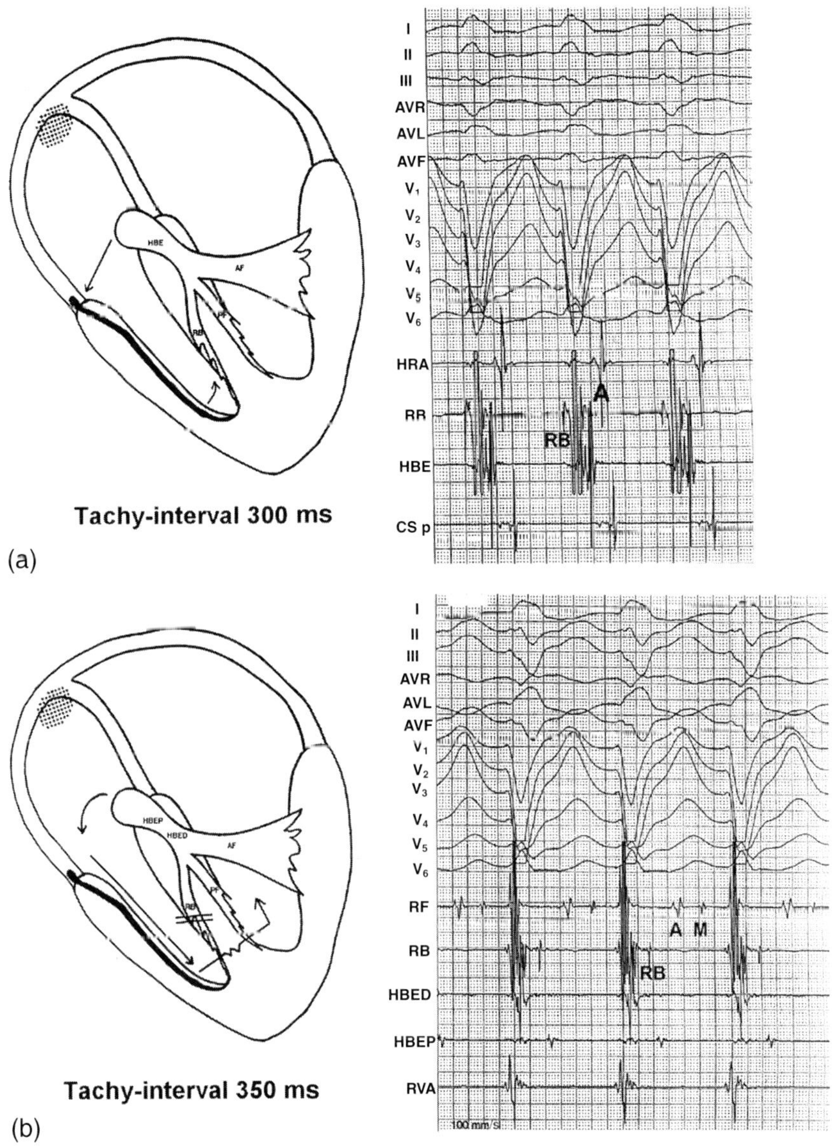

Figure 3.11 (a) A typical short VH (V-RB) antidromic tachycardia with anterograde conduction over an atriofascicular pathway. (b) In the same patient, on occurrence of a retrograde RBBB, the intracavitary recording shows a long V-RB tachycardia, where the RBB potential is recorded after the QRS complex, and the tachycardia cycle length increases. Note that the frontal plane QRS axis also changes (see text).

antidromic tachycardia also favors a longer distance between the distal accessory pathway and the distal Purkinje fibers. The same reasoning holds for the V-RB interval: a longer interval with a less early recording of the QRS. However, one has to be careful in case of a retrograde RBBB (sometimes a transient phenomenon and not necessarily coupled with an anterograde RBBB). In that

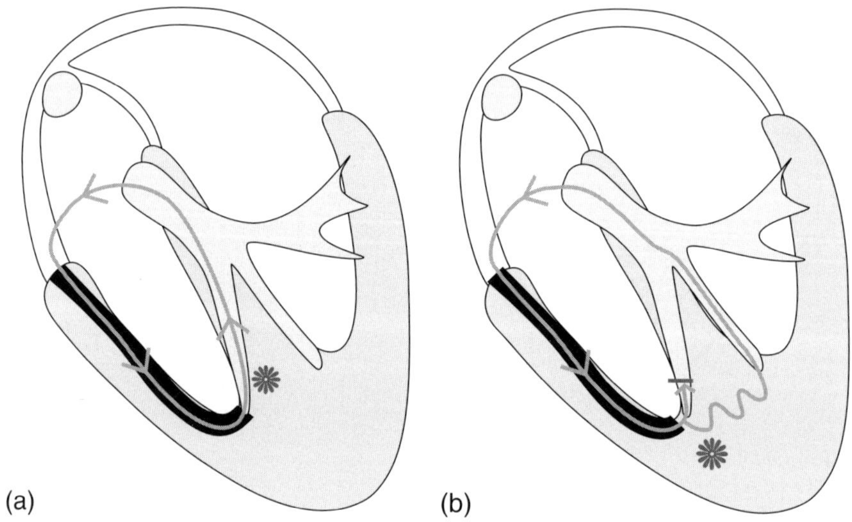

Figure 3.12 Illustration showing the proposed explanation for the frontal plane QRS axis shift during preexcited tachycardia with anterograde conduction over an atriofascicular pathway observed after retrograde RBBB (with a long V-H interval) depicted in Fig. 3.13. Asterisk marks the change in the exit point of the activation wavefront that will depolarize the right ventricle.

situation, the V-RB (and V-His) will be significantly longer because of transseptal activation of the left bundle branch, in spite of the presence of an atriofascicular pathway (Fig. 3.11).

2 We have reported RF catheter ablation at the distal end (targeting a distal "M" potential) with preservation of the right bundle potential and absence of a right bundle–branch block in spite of 2 minutes of current application at that site, as well as the modification of the QRS complexes during tachycardia after the first RF pulse (Figs. 3.15 and 3.16), suggesting not only a direct myocardial connection but also distal myocardial arborization of this pathway [45].

3 RF current application at the distal "M" potential would most likely cause automatic activity with a similar QRS morphology as during overt preexcitation. However, it will be difficult to rule out a ventricular origin of such a rhythm, weakening such an argument.

Response to AV nodal blocking agents

The atriofascicular pathway is an AV node-like structure and as sensitive to intravenous adenosine as the AV node itself. The usual response to adenosine is a transient block both at the AV nodal level and in the atriofascicular pathway [46]. It has been reported that atriofascicular pathways are less sensitive to intravenous verapamil than the AV node. We use it to challenge our patients, after RF catheter ablation, to assess recurrence of conduction through the decremental pathway, which is sometimes impossible to evaluate on

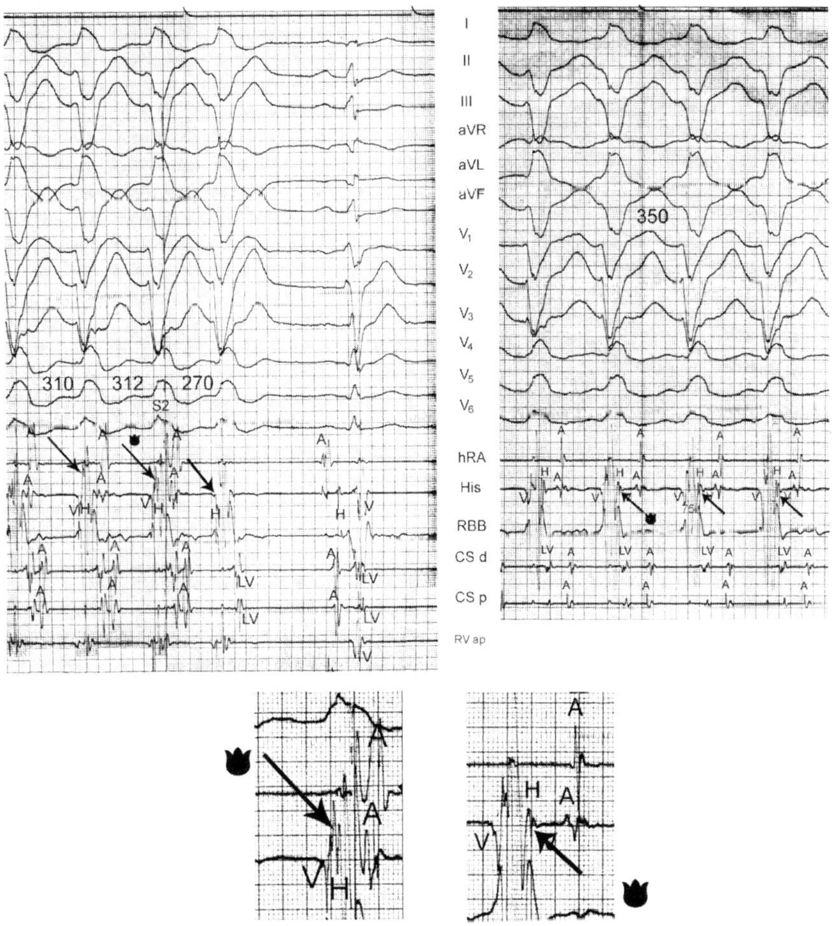

Figure 3.13 (a) Preexcited tachycardia with a short VH interval and a cycle length around 310 ms. A late lateral right atrial premature beat advances RV activation and terminates tachycardia because of VA block. (b) The same patient during RBBB showing a longer tachycardia cycle length (350 ms) due to prolongation of the VH and VA conduction time. (c, d) Enlarged views of the His bundle potentials during short and long VH tachycardia (black tulips).

the baseline 12-lead ECG. Verapamil will expose preexcitation during sinus rhythm (Fig. 3.17) in case of recurrence of conduction through the atriofascicular fiber, although it lacks efficacy in terminating circus movement tachycardia [47].

Mapping and RF catheter ablation

Some features are unique to atriofascicular fibers. Mapping of the atrial insertion during ventricular stimulation is usually not possible because these decrementally conducting pathways usually do not conduct retrogradely. Eccentric VA conduction if present should be a clue to the presence of associated

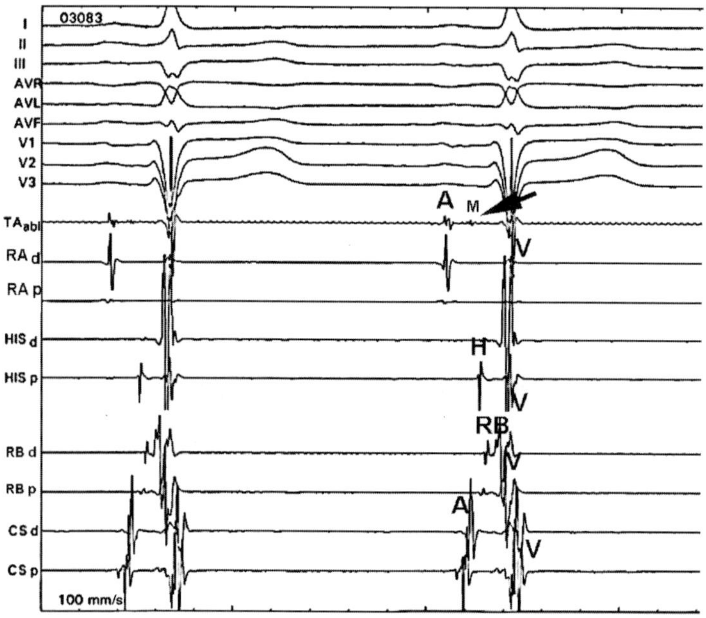

(a)

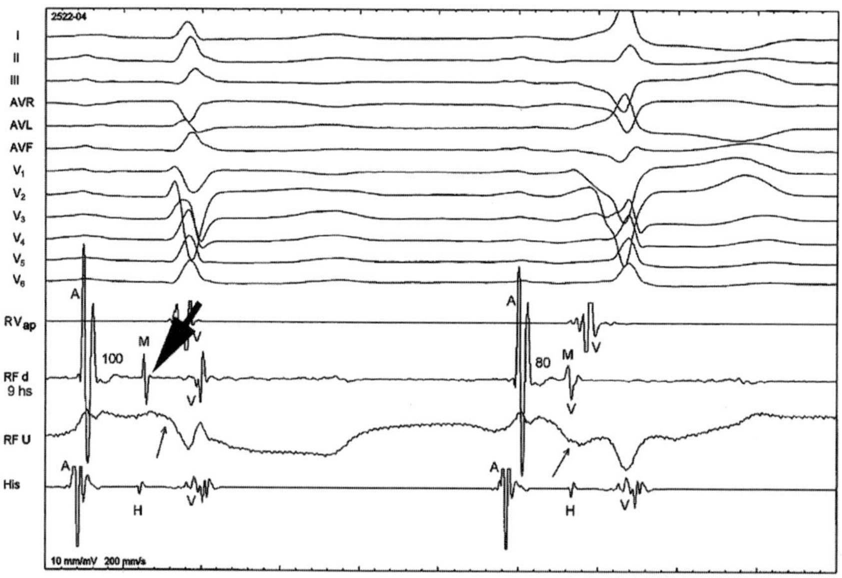

(b)

Figure 3.14 Two examples of an "M" potential (black arrowheads). (a) There is a high-frequency and low-amplitude accessory pathway potential recorded from an ablation catheter, located at the right lateral tricuspid annulus, in a patient with an atriofascicular pathway. Successful catheter ablation was carried out at this site. (b) A high-frequency and high-amplitude "M" potential was recorded in the setting of intermittent conduction over a short AV Mahaim fiber (see Chapter 8).

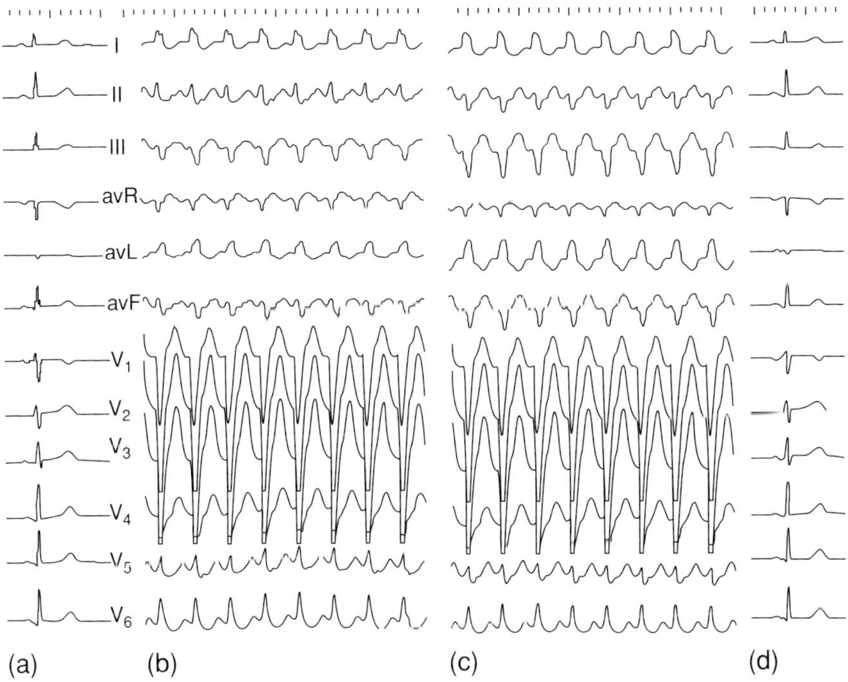

Figure 3.15 The 12-lead ECG (a) before catheter ablation, (b) during antidromic tachycardia, (c) during antidromic tachycardia after the first episode of RF current, and (d) after successful catheter ablation, without RBBB. Paper speed: 25 mm/s.

rapidly conducting bypass tracts. A short AV fiber can be located by mapping the site of the earliest ventricular activation at the annulus, as with other anterogradely conducting accessory AV pathways. In atriofascicular pathways or long AV fibers the distal (nonannular) insertion cannot be mapped in this way. In addition, these decremental pathways are unusually sensitive to mechanical trauma. Accidentally touching the annulus with the ablation catheter can result in transient abolition of conduction through the pathway, lasting minutes to hours [35]. The following strategies have been used to overcome these problems:

1 Searching for the "M" potential (Fig. 3.14) along the tricuspid annulus is the gold standard technique. The ablation catheter should be moved cautiously along the annulus avoiding bumps to the Mahaim tissue. The potential may be as large as the His bundle potential or small and narrow with low amplitude. Catheter ablation at a site with an "M" potential is likely to be successful. Automatic rhythms (Mahaim automatic tachycardia [MAT]) are observed during RF current delivery in most patients with Mahaim fibers (see Chapter 8). It is probably due to heat-related automaticity of nodelike tissue as is also seen during slow AV nodal pathway ablation. MAT is in most cases short-lived but may sometimes last up to 2 minutes. At least in some patients it is necessary to completely terminate those rhythms to prevent recurrences.

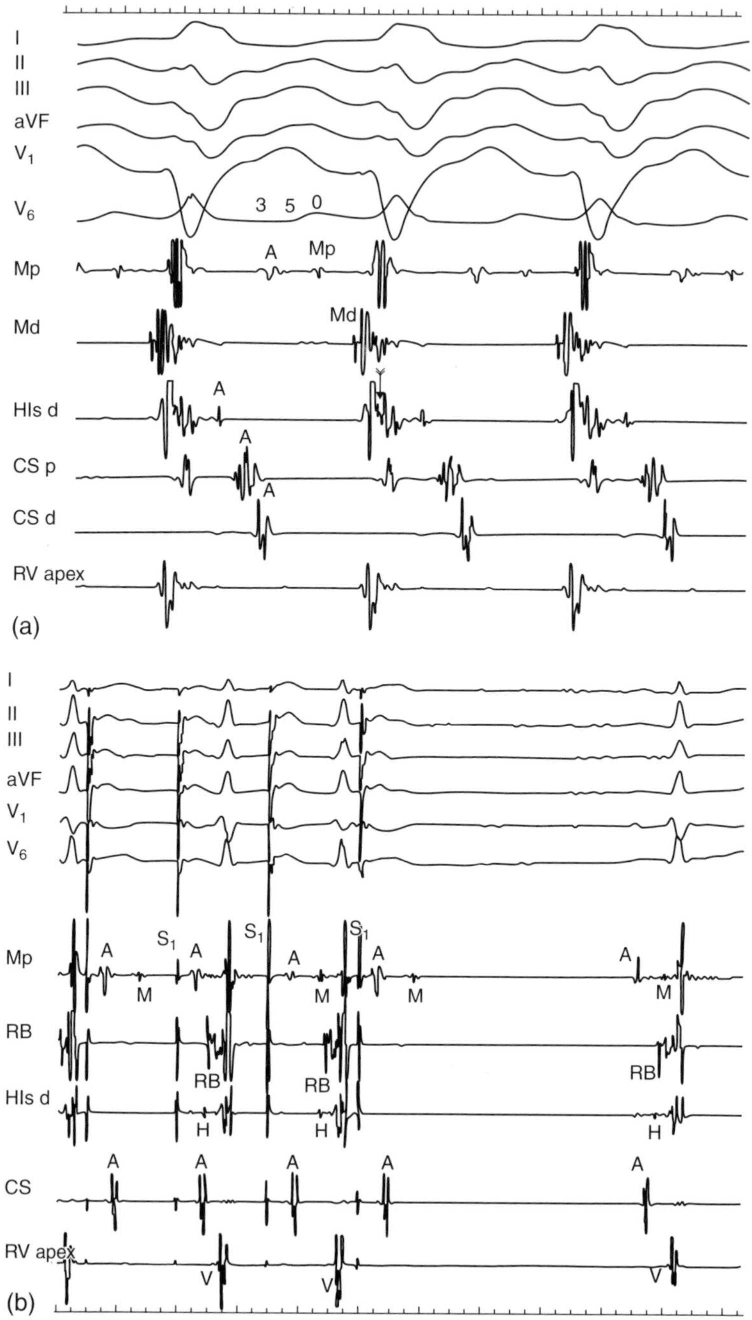

Figure 3.16 (a) Antidromic AV tachycardia over a Mahaim (M) fiber. The distal M potential precedes The QRS complex by 10 ms. Retrograde conduction occurs over the AV node His-Purkinje system. The anterograde distal M potential is recorded 6 ms earlier than the retrograde right bundle potential (which precedes the QRS complex by 4 ms). Paper speed: 200 mm/s. (b) Right atrial pacing after successful catheter ablation aimed at the distal insertion of the Mahaim fiber. There is Wenckebach block at the AV node level with simultaneous conduction through the proximal part of the Mahaim fiber (AM potential interval), but complete conduction block inside this long Mahaim fiber. Paper speed: 100 mm/s.

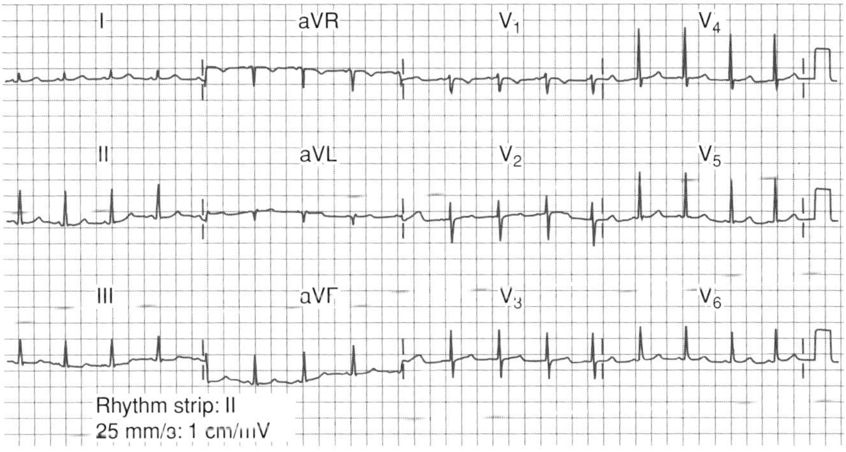

(a)

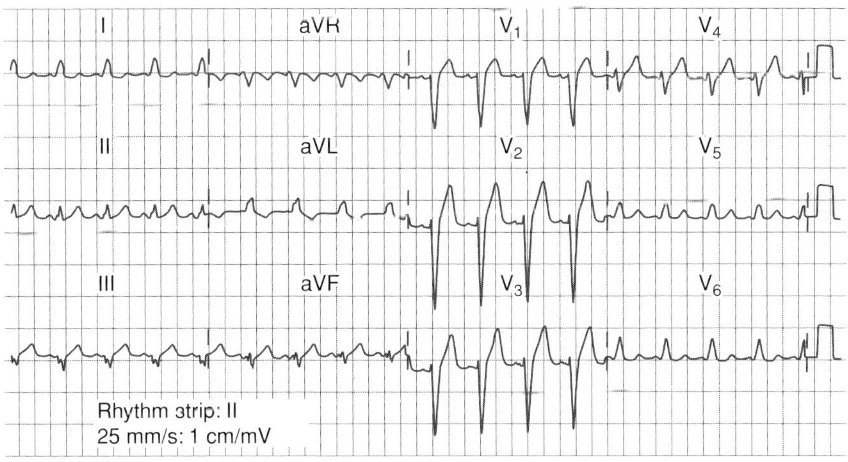

(b)

Figure 3.17 (a) A 12-lead ECG in a patient with an atriofascicular pathway. There is no minimal preexcitation (qR pattern in lead III). (b) An ECG that was done 5 minutes after an intravenous bolus of 5 mg of verapamil. The PR interval did not change, but an overt preexcitation is evident, and it is consistent with a right posterolateral accessory pathway (successful RF catheter ablation was carried out at the tricuspid annulus at 9 o'clock in LAO projection).

2 Other methods like finding the shortest stimulus-to-QRS interval by pacing at different atrial sites close to the annulus, or the extrastimulus mapping technique, trying to find the longest coupling interval from an atrial premature beat causing resetting during circus movement tachycardia, or looking for the greatest amount of advancement of the next QRS complex using a fixed coupling interval are time-consuming and inaccurate methods of mapping.

Arrhythmias related to decrementally conducting AV or atriofascicular fibers

1 Antidromic tachycardia with anterograde conduction over a long fiber;
2 AVNRT with bystander Mahaim conduction;
3 Spontaneous fast automatic tachycardia arising in the decrementally conducting fiber;
4 Spontaneous slow automatic rhythm arising in the decrementally conducting fiber;
5 Automaticity induced by RF ablation at the site of atrial insertion of the fiber;
6 Atrial fibrillation with anterograde conduction over the decrementally conducting fiber;
7 Nonreentrant preexcited tachycardia due to simultaneous dual conduction. Over the decrementally conducting fiber.

Antidromic tachycardia with anterograde conduction over a long decrementally conducting fiber

This is the most common type of tachycardia associated with decrementally conducting fibers (Fig. 3.6). The tachycardia is usually regular with a mean cycle length of 309 ± 52 milliseconds (range 220–450). The QRS complex width is usually around 0, 13 ± 0.01 seconds (range 0.11–0.15) and shows a-LBBB-like configuration with a smooth slope of the downstroke in V_1 and a frontal plane axis between 0° and −75°. In rare cases of an anteriorly located fiber the axis can be around +60°. The QRS width during tachycardia is related to the distal site of insertion of the fiber. The closer to the right bundle branch exit, the narrower the QRS. Retrograde VA conduction over the normal conduction system is associated with a time interval between 100 and 140 milliseconds. The retrograde P wave usually cannot be recognized because it falls within the final portion of the QRS complex. The major differential diagnosis is an SVT (orthodromic AV reentrant tachycardia using an AV bypass tract retrogradely or rarely an AVNRT with LBBB) [20].

AVNRT with bystander conduction over a decrementally conducting fiber

AVNRT is found in a patient with a Mahaim fiber in up to 10% of the patients [48–50]. It can occur as a narrow QRS tachycardia, usually with a faster rate than the antidromic reciprocating tachycardia, or it can present as an arrhythmia showing ventricular preexcitation by bystander anterograde conduction over the fiber (Figs. 3.18 and 3.19). The QRS complex would be indistinguishable from the real antidromic reciprocating tachycardia because anterograde AV conduction goes over the fiber. The finding of fusion beats during tachycardia (usually at induction) is the major clue to diagnose such a mechanism. During the electrophysiologic study block in the accessory pathway can be achieved by atrial or ventricular premature stimuli (Fig. 3.19). Sometimes no spontaneous or induced fusion beats can be seen, and the diagnosis of bystander anterograde Mahaim conduction can only be made when AVNRT with the same rate can be induced after ablation of the fiber [51].

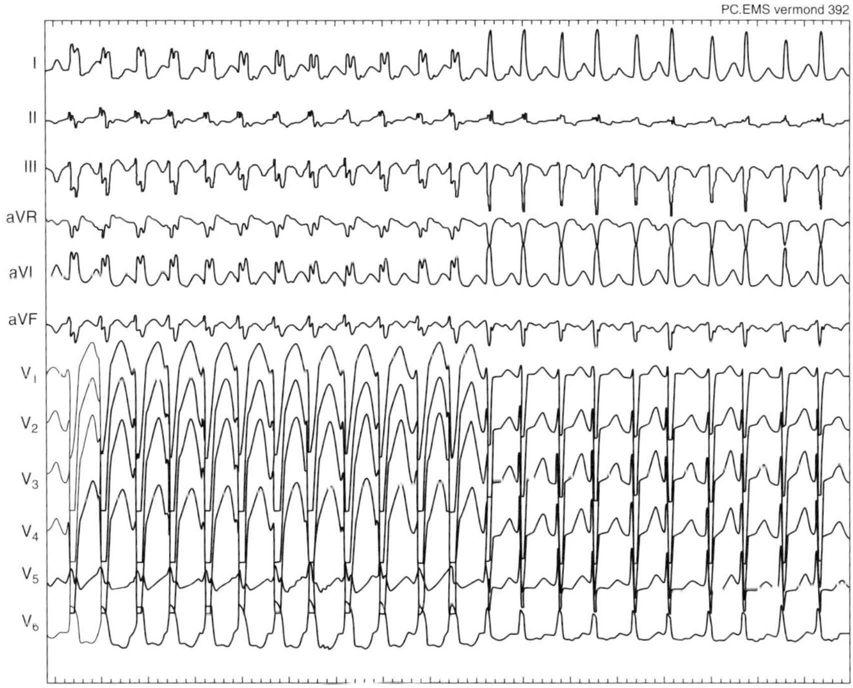

Figure 3.18 A LBBB tachycardia is induced during atrial pacing. Atrial pacing before the tachycardia showed a normal PR interval and a minimally preexcited QRS (rS pattern in lead III and absence of q waves in the left-sided leads).

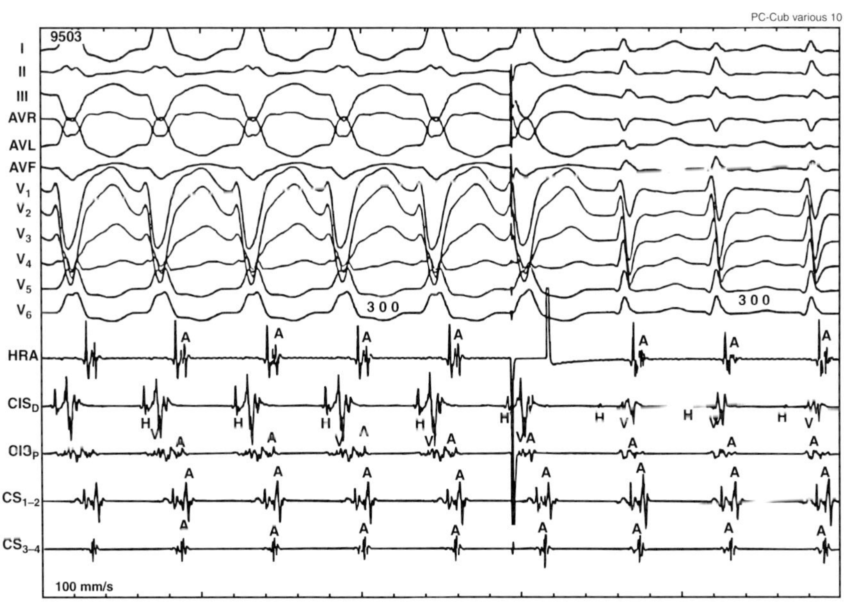

Figure 3.19 The same patient as in Fig. 3.16. A late right atrial premature beat delivered at the right lateral wall, blocks in the atriofascicular fiber without resetting the next atrial (A) or His potential. The intracavitary recordings are consistent with AVNRT.

Spontaneous automatic tachycardia arising in a decrementally conducting fiber

Spontaneous automaticity arising in the decrementally conducting fiber has been described occasionally [9]. The clinical presentation of such rhythms can be as premature beats in a bigeminal pattern, as slow rhythms resembling accelerated idioventricular rhythm, or as fast nonsustained bursts of repetitive tachycardia. We have seen 2 patients with frequent episodes of repetitive automatic rhythms as the presenting arrhythmia, without a true antidromic tachycardia. There was no VA conduction over the AV node and over the atriofascicular fiber (Fig. 3.20). The QRS complex morphology during tachycardia equals the one during atrial pacing at the same rate. Patients having spontaneous automaticity associated with decrementally conducting fibers are younger (15 ± 7 yr) than patients (26 ± 13 yr) without spontaneous automaticity [52].

Spontaneous slow automatic rhythm arising in a decrementally conducting fiber

Spontaneous slow automaticity arising in decrementally conducting fibers is an infrequent rhythm that was present in only 7.5% (3 out of 40) of our patients. Those rhythms are clinically silent (Fig. 3.21) resembling an AIVR (accelerated idioventricular rhythm). In 2 of our 3 patients, spontaneously occurring automatic beats triggered episodes of antidromic tachycardia (Fig. 8.4, Chapter 8). Automaticity was abolished after successful catheter ablation of the decrementally conducting fiber. In both patients it was required to terminate all heat-induced MAT [15, 52] to abolish conduction over and spontaneous decrementally conducting fiber automaticity.

Automaticity induced during RF ablation at the atrial insertion of the decrementally conducting fiber

Heat-induced automaticity is a long-known phenomenon occurring when ablating the slow AV nodal pathway in patients with AVNRT. Some authors believe that heating the compact node at a distance is the most likely explanation [53]. Others believe that it is caused by heating AV nodal tissue at the posterior extension of the AV node. It is also known that regular atrial or ventricular myocardium does not generate such automaticity. The observation of automaticity during ablation of Mahaim fibers (MAT) was reported in the early nineties. McClelland *et al.* [13] found it in 11 out of 23 patients, Heald *et al.* [14] found it in 12 out of 16 patients and called it "stuttering block," and Braun *et al.* [54] found it in 15 out of 15 patients. We found it in 30 out of 33 patients, during ablation at the tricuspid annulus targeting the Mahaim "compact node." MAT usually starts immediately or a couple of seconds after current delivery. Automaticity may be short-lived, as short as four beats, or very long-lasting up to 90 seconds (see Fig. 9.5, p. 136). The attitude toward the occurrence of MAT changed from the previous concern about stability of the catheter [55] to a desirable event meaning a hallmark of successful ablation. We believe that in some cases with prolonged automaticity, sometimes associated

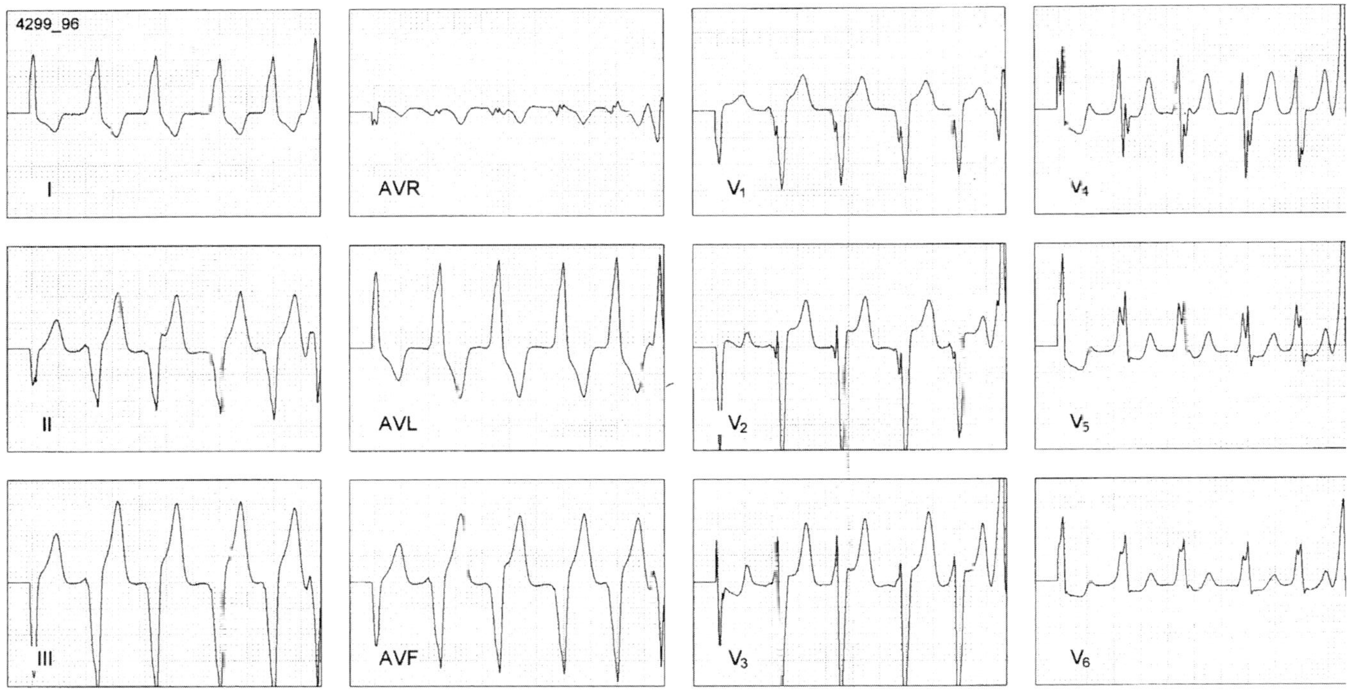

Figure 3.20 A 12-lead ECG shows a slow LBBB-like tachycardia (QRS = 0.12 s) with AV dissociation, irregular RR intervals and a cycle length between 400 and 480 ms. The frontal plane QRS axis is -50°.

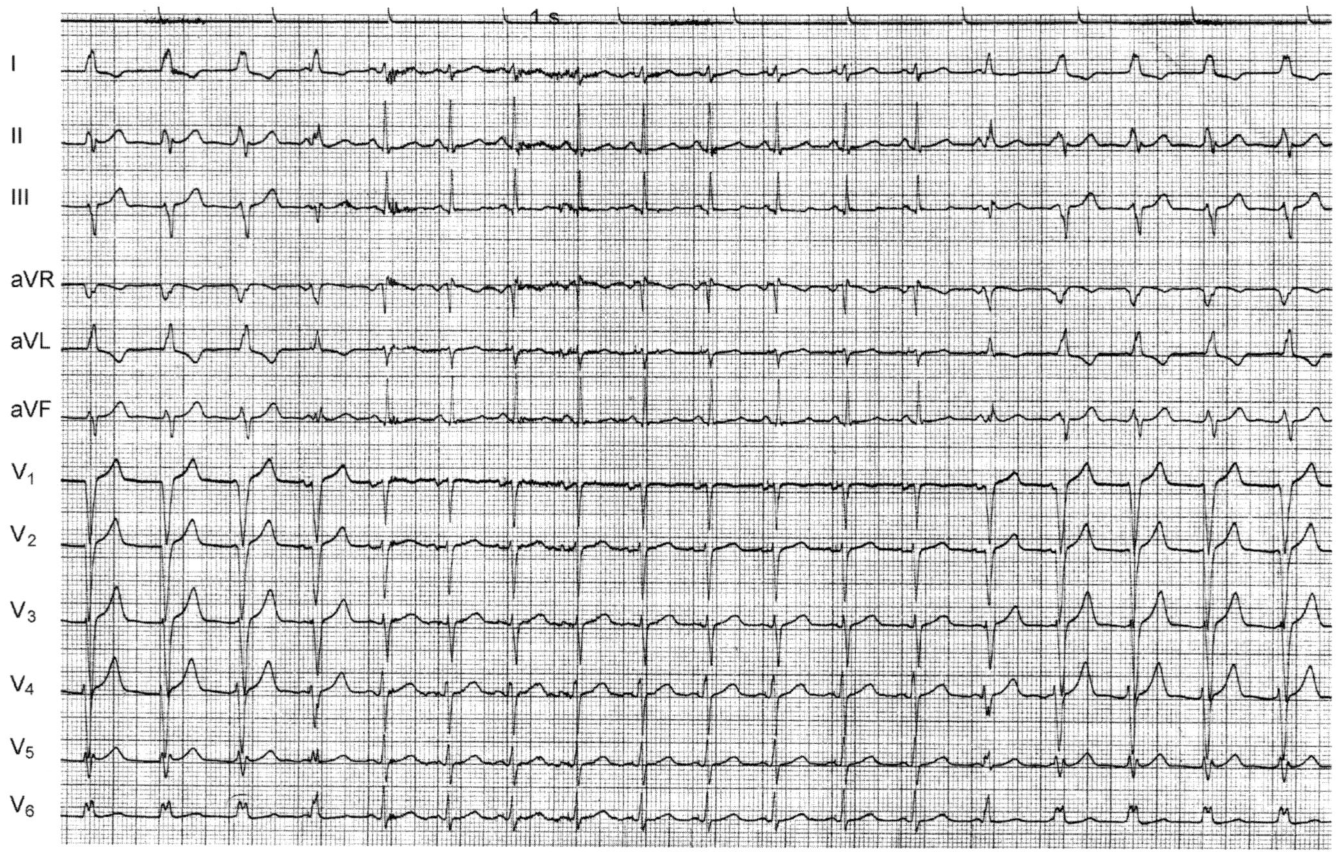

Figure 3.21 A 12-lead ECG showing sinus rhythm (580 ms) between two episodes of Mahaim automaticity (640 ms); 4th and 14th QRS complexes are fusion beats.

with spontaneous automatic rhythms, complete termination of MAT may be required for a long-term successful outcome.

Atrial fibrillation with anterograde conduction over the decrementally conducting pathway

We saw spontaneous atrial fibrillation as the presenting arrhythmia in patients with Mahaim fibers only once in 40 patients. It was a 50-year-old patient (Fig. 3.22) without retrograde conduction over the fiber. After successful ablation of the atriofascicular fiber atrial fibrillation did not recur during a follow-up of 2.5 years. Miller *et al.* [51] ablated a Mahaim fiber during atrial fibrillation. After ablation atrial fibrillation could not be re-induced. We reviewed 14 articles [13, 14, 16, 18, 19, 22, 48, 51, 54, 57–60] with a total of 208 patients with Mahaim fibers, and only 4 patients had atrial fibrillation as the presenting arrhythmia (1.9%). It is a much lower incidence as compared with the 32% incidence of atrial fibrillation in patients with the Wolff-Parkinson-White (WPW) syndrome [61]. Degeneration of circus movement tachycardia to atrial fibrillation was the mechanism in 25% of the patients with WPW, studied by Bauernfeind *et al.* [62]. This mechanism may explain atrial fibrillation in the patient of Brugada *et al.* [60], who had an additional right posteroseptal AP and antidromic tachycardia, but can not explain atrial fibrillation in our patient who did not have other arrhythmias. The reason for the small incidence

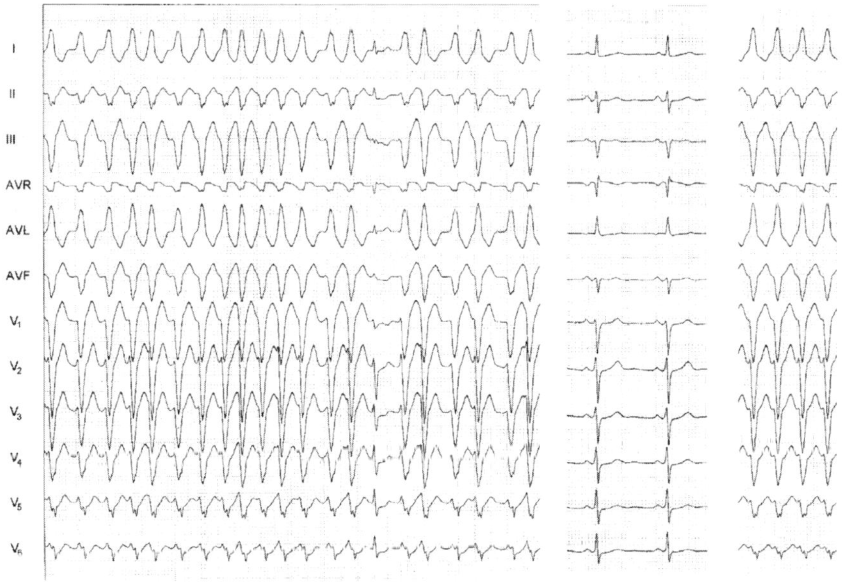

(a) (b) (c)

Figure 3.22 (a) Atrial fibrillation in a patient with an atriofascicular fiber. QRS pattern is similar to QRS during atrial pacing (c). (b) Sinus rhythm with minimal preexcitation with an rS pattern in lead III.

of atrial fibrillation in patients with decrementally conducting fibers remains unknown, but the presence of the Mahaim fiber itself seems to be important, as in the case reported by Miller *et al.*, where atrial fibrillation could not be re-induced after ablation of the fiber.

Nonreentrant preexcited tachycardia due to simultaneous dual conduction in a decrementally conducting fiber

Nonreentrant SVT with simultaneous conduction over the fast and slow AV nodal pathway has been widely reported [63]. These patients share some common features. They are usually refractory to antiarrhythmic drug treatment. Tachycardia can be aggravated by the use of drugs. In the majority of patients no reentrant AV nodal tachycardia can be induced. The effective refractory period of the "fast" pathway is shorter than the "slow" pathway; they usually show absence of retrograde VA conduction. Without retrograde conduction over the "slow" pathway at the time of anterograde conduction over the "fast" pathway, conduction can proceed over the "slow" pathway and with a critical atrial cycle length it can reach the ventricle a second time. We have recently

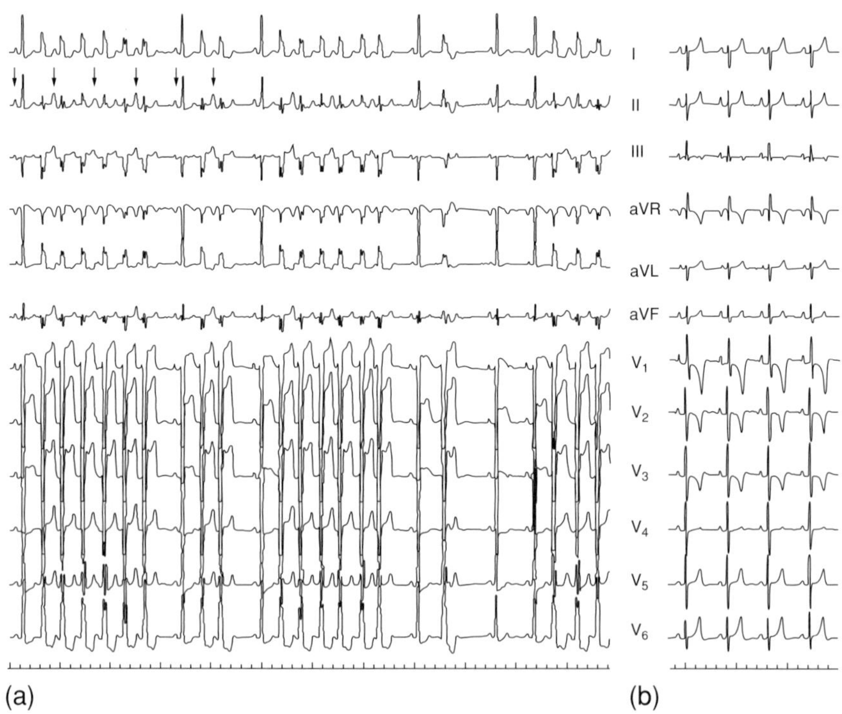

Figure 3.23 (a) A 12-lead ECG during sinus rhythm showing frequent episodes of nonsustained tachycardia based on one sinus P wave resulting into two QRS complexes. Sinus P waves are indicated by arrows. Note that an episode of tachycardia terminates because of block in the "slow" decrementally conducting pathway. The QRS complex after the pause is a fusion complex between AV conduction over the AV node and the atriofascicular fiber. (b) The ECG after catheter ablation of the fiber. Paperspeed: 25 mm/s.

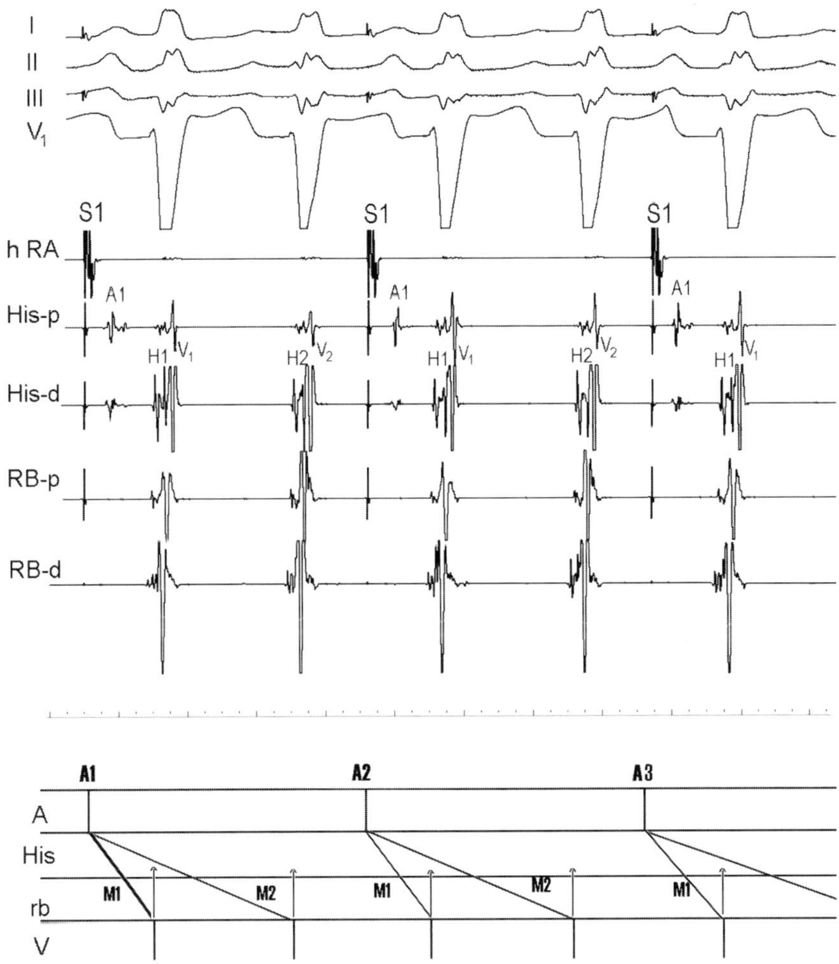

Figure 3.24 High right atrial pacing at 800 ms with a 1:2 P/QRS response. There is reversal of the normal His bundle–right bundle sequence (see arrow in the ladder diagram at the bottom). Paperspeed: 150 mm/s.

reported [64] a patient with atriofascicular fiber showing likewise characteristics: an incessant tachycardia due to a 1:2 P/QRS relationship (Figs. 3.23 and 3.24), no reentrant antidromic tachycardia could be induced. The tachycardia did not respond to antiarrhythmic drugs (sotalol and amiodarone), and the patient did not have VA conduction through the fiber. No further dual conduction occurred after successful catheter ablation of the decremental pathway.

References

1 Mahaim I, Bennett. Nouvelle recherches sur les connexions superieures de la branche gauche du faisceau de His-Tawara avec cloison interventriculaire. *Cardiologia* 1938;1:61.

2 Becker AE, Anderson RH. The anatomical substrates of Wolff–Parkinson–White syndrome: a clinico-pathologic correlation in seven patients. *Circulation* 1978;57:870.

3 Anderson RH, Becker AE. Stanley Kent and accessory atrioventricular connections. *J Thoracic Cardiovasc Surg* 1981;81:649.
4 Guiraudon CM, Guiraudon GM, Klein GJ. Histologic evidence for an accessory atrioventricular pathway with AV-node-like morphology. *Circulation* 1988;78 (suppl 2):40.
5 Klein GJ, Guiraudon GM, Kerr CR, *et al.* "Nodoventricular" accessory pathway: evidence for a distinct accessory atrioventricular pathway with atrioventricular node-like properties. *J Am Coll Cardiol* 1988;11:1035.
6 Peinado R, Merino JL, Ramírez L, *et al.* Decremental atriofascicular accessory pathway with bidirectional conduction: delineation of atrial and ventricular insertion by radiofrequency current application. *J Cardiovascular Electrophysiol* 2001;12:489.
7 Hluchy J, Schickel S, Jörger U, *et al.* Electrophysiologic characteristics and radiofrequency ablation of concealed nodofascicular and left anterograde atriofascicular pathways. *J Cardiovasc Electrophysiol* 2000;11:211.
8 Gallagher JJ, Smith WM, Kassell JH, *et al.* Role of Mahaim fibers in cardiac arrhythmias in man. *Circulation* 1981;64:176.
9 Sosa E, Scanavacca M. Repetitive nonsustained wide QRS complex tachycardia: what is the tachycardia mechanism? *J Cardiovasc Electrophysiol* 2001;12:977.
10 Wellens HJJ. Electrical Stimulation of the heart in the study and treatment of tachycardias. Baltimore: University Park Press; 1971.
11 Tchou P, Lehmann MH, Jazayeri M, *et al.* Atriofascicular connection or a nodoventricular Mahaim fiber? Electrophysiologic elucidation of the pathway and associated reentrant circuit. *Circulation* 1988;77:837.
12 Porkolab F, Alpert B, Scheinman MM. Failure of atrial premature beats to reset atriofascicular tachycardia. *Pacing Clin Electrophysiol* 1999;22:528.
13 McClelland JH, Wang X, Beckman KJ, *et al.* Radiofrequency catheter ablation of right atriofascicular (Mahaim) accessory pathways guided by accessory pathway activation potentials. *Circulation* 1994;89:2655.
14 Heald SC, Davies DW, Ward DE, *et al.* Radiofrequency catheter ablation of Mahaim tachycardia by targeting Mahaim potentials at the tricuspid annulus. *Br Heart J* 1995;73:250.
15 Sternick EB, Gerken LM, Vrandecic MO. Appraisal of "Mahaim" automatic tachycardia. *J Cardiovasc Electrophysiol* 2002;13:244.
16 Bardy GH, Fedor JM, German LD, *et al.* Surface electrocardiographic clues suggesting presence of a nodofascicular Mahaim fiber. *J Am Coll Cardiol* 1984;3:1161.
17 Ellenbogen KA, Ramirez NM, Packer DL, *et al.* Accessory nodoventricular (Mahaim) fibers. A clinical review. *Pacing Clin Electrophysiol* 1986;9:868.
18 Haissaguerre M, Cauchemez B, Marcus F, *et al.* Characteristics of the ventricular insertion sites of accessory pathways with anterograde decremental conduction properties. *Circulation* 1995;91:1077.
19 Sternick EB, Timmermans C, Sosa E, *et al.* The electrocardiogram during sinus rhythm and tachycardia in patients with anterograde conduction over Mahaim fibers. The importance of an "rS" pattern in lead III. *J Am Coll Cardiol* 2004;44:1626.
20 Sternick EB, Cruz Filho FE, Timmermans C, *et al.* The electrocardiogram during tachycardia in patients with anterograde conduction over a Mahaim fiber. Old criteria revisited. *Heart Rhythm* 2004;1:406
21 Sternick EB. Role of Mahaim fibers in cardiac arrhythmias. Maastricht, The Netherlands: Datawyse, Universitaire pers Maastricht; 2004.
22 Klein LS, Hackett K, Zipes DP, *et al.* Radiofrequency catheter ablation of Mahaim fibers at the tricuspid annulus. *Circulation* 1993;87:738.
23 Shimizu A, Ohe T, Takaki H, *et al.* Narrow QRS complex tachycardia with atrioventricular dissociation. *Pacing Clin Electrophysiol* 1988;11:384.

24 Mittleman RS, Huang SKS. Ablation of Mahaim fibers. In: Huang SKS, ed. *Radiofrequency Catheter Ablation of Cardiac Arrhythmias. Basic Concepts and Clinical Application*. Armonk, NY: Futura Publishing; 1995:352.
25 Josephson ME. Preexcitation syndromes. In: *Clinical Cardiac Electrophysiology. Techniques and Interpretations*. Philadelphia, USA: Lippincott Williams & Wilkins; 2002:404.
26 Ott P, Marcus FI. Familial Mahaim Syndrome. *Ann Noninvas Eletrocardiol* 2001;6:272.
27 Gmeiner R, Keung CK, Hammer I, *et al*. Tachycardia caused by an accessory nodoventricular tract: a clinico-pathologic correlation. *Eur Heart J* 1984;5:233.
28 Davidson NC, Morton JB, Sanders P, *et al*. Latent Mahaim fiber as a cause of antidromic reciprocating tachycardia: recognition and successful radiofrequency ablation. *J Cardiovasc Electrophysiol* 2002;13:74.
29 Bogun F, Kalusche D, Li YG, *et al*. Septal Q waves in surface electrocardiographic lead V6 exclude minimal ventricular preexcitation. *Am J Cardiol* 1999;84:101.
30 Tranchesi J, Moffa PJ. *Electrocardiograma Normal e Patológico*. São Paulo, SP: Atheneu Editora LTDA; 1983:86.
31 Pileggi F, Tranchesi J, Grandisky B, *et al*. Análise vectorcardiográfica da ativação ventricular em indivíduos com eletrocardiograma do tipo S1 S2 S3. *Arq Bras Cardiol* 1961;14:373.
32 Miller JM, Olgin JE. Catheter ablation of free-wall accessory pathways and "Mahaim" fibers. In: Zipes DP, Haissaguerre M, eds. *Catheter Ablation of Cardiac Arrhythmias*, 2nd ed. Armonk, NY: Futura Publishing; 2002:277.
33 His RG, Lamb LE. Electrocardiographic findings in 122,043 individuals. *Circulation* 1962;25:947.
34 Haissaguerre M, Warin JF, Le Metayer P, *et al*. Catheter ablation of Mahaim fibers with preservation of atrioventricular nodal conduction. *Circulation* 1990;82:418.
35 Cappato R, Schluter M, Weiss C, *et al*. Catheter-induced mechanical conduction block of right-sided accessory fibers with Mahaim-type preexcitation to guide radiofrequency ablation. *Circulation* 1994;90:282.
36 Fung WHJ, Chan HCK, Chan WWL, Sanderson JE. Ablation of the Mahaim Pathway guided by noncontact mapping. *J Cardiovasc Electrophysiol* 2002;13:1064.
37 Tan HL, Wittkampf FHM, Nakagawa H, Derksen R. Atriofascicular accessory pathway. *J Cardiovasc Electrophysiol* 2004;15:118.
38 Cosio FG, Anderson RH, Kuck KH, *et al*. ESCWGA/NASPE/P Experts consensus statement. Living anatomy of the atrioventricular junctions. A guide to electrophysiologic mapping. *J Cardiovasc Electrophysiol* 1999;10:1162.
39 Wyndham CRC, Smith T, Meeran MK, *et al*. Epicardial activation in patients with left bundle branch block. *Circulation* 1980;61:696.
40 Vassalo JA, Cassidy DM, Marchlinski F, *et al*. Endocardial activation of the left bundle branch block. *Circulation* 1984;69:914.
41 Rodriguez LM, Timmermans C, Nabar A, *et al*. Variable patterns of septal activation in patients with left bundle branch block and heart failure. *J Cardiovasc Electrophysiol* 2003;14:135.
42 Kuck KH, Brugada P, Wellens HJJ. Observations on the antidromic type of circus movement tachycardia in the Wolff–Parkinson–White syndrome. *J Am Coll Cardiol* 1983;2:1003.
43 Sternick EB, Timmermans C, Rodriguez LM, *et al*. Effect of right bundle branch block on antidromic circus movement tachycardia in patients with presumed atriofascicular pathways. *J Cardiovasc Electrophysiol* (in press).
44 Mounsey JP, Griffith MJ, McComb JM. Radiofrequency ablation of a Mahaim fiber following localization of Mahaim pathway potentials. *J Cardiovasc Electrophysiol* 1994;5:432.
45 Sternick EB, Timmermans C, Rodriguez LM, Wellens HJJ. Mahaim fiber: an atriofascicular or a long atrioventricular pathway? *Heart Rhythm* 2004;1:724.

46 Ellenbogen KA, Rogers R, Old W. Pharmacological characterization of conduction over a Mahaim fiber: evidence for adenosine sensitive conduction. *Pacing Clin Electrophysiol* 1989;12:1396.

47 Strasberg B, Coelho A, Palileo E, *et al.* Pharmacological observations in patients with nodoventricular pathways. *Br Heart J* 1984;51:84

48 Grogin HR, Lee RJ, Kwasman M, Epstein LM, *et al.* Radiofrequency catheter ablation of atriofascicular and nodoventricular Mahaim tracts. *Circulation* 1994;90:272.

49 Bardy GH, German LD, Packer DL, *et al.* Mechanism of tachycardia using a nodoventricular Mahaim fiber. *Am J Cardiol* 1984;54:1140.

50 De Ponti R, Storti C, Stanke A, *et al.* Radiofrequency catheter ablation in patients with Mahaim-type slow conduction accessory right atrio-ventricular pathway. *Cardiologia* 1994; 39:169.

51 Miller JM, Harper GR, Rothman SA, Hsia HH. Radiofrequency catheter ablation of an atriofascicular pathway during atrial fibrillation. A case report. *J Cardiovasc Electrophysiol* 1994;5:846.

52 Sternick EB, Timmermans C, Sosa E, *et al.* Automaticity in Mahaim fibers. *J Cardiovasc Electrophysiol* 2004;15:738.

53 Thibault B, de Bakker JMT, Hocini M, *et al.* Origin of heat induced accelerated junctional rhythm. *J Cardiovasc Electrophysiol* 1998;9:631.

54 Braun E, Siebbels J, Volkmer M, *et al.* Radiofrequency-induced preexcited automatic rhythm during ablation accessory pathways with Mahaim-type preexcitation: does it predicts clinical outcome? *Pacing Clin Electrophysiol* 1997;20:1121.

55 Davies DW. Treatment of "Mahaim" tachycardias by radiofrequency catheter ablation. In: Camm J, Lindemans FW, eds. *Transvenous Defibrillation and Radiofrequency Ablation.* Armonk, NY: Futura Publishing; 1995:199.

56 Kottkamp H, Hindricks G, Shenasa H, *et al.* Variants of preexcitation-specialized atriofascicular pathways, nodofascicular pathways, and fasciculoventricular pathways: electrophysiologic findings and target sites for radiofrequency catheter ablation. *J Cardiovasc Electrophysiol* 1996;7:916.

57 Ellenbogen KA, Ramirez NM, Packer DL, *et al.* Accessory nodoventricular (Mahaim) fibers. A clinical review. *Pacing Clin Electrophysiol* 1986;9:868.

58 Bockeria LA, Chigogidze NA, Golukhova EZ, Artjukhina TV. Diagnosis and surgical treatment of tachycardias in patients with nodoventricular fibers. *Pacing Clin Electrophysiol* 1991;14:2004.

59 Okishige K, Friedman PL. New observations on decremental atriofascicular and nodofascicular fibers: implications for catheter ablation. *Pacing Clin Electrophysiol* 1995;18:986.

60 Brugada J, Sanchez JM, Kuzmicic B, *et al.* Radiofrequency catheter ablation of atriofascicular accessory pathways guided by discrete electrical potentials recorded at the tricuspid annulus. *Pacing Clin Electrophysiol* 1995;18:1388.

61 Campbell RWF, Smith RA, Gallagher JJ, *et al.* Atrial fibrillation in the pre-excitation syndrome. *Am J Cardiol* 1977;40:514.

62 Bauernfeind RA, Wyndham CR, Swiryn SP, *et al.* Paroxysmal atrial fibrillation in the Wolff-Parkinson-White syndrome. *Am J Cardiol* 1981;47:562.

63 Csapo G. Paroxysmal nonreentrant tachycardia due to simultaneous conduction through dual atrioventricular nodal pathways. *Am J Cardiol* 1979;43:1033.

64 Sternick EB, Sosa E, Scanavacca M, Wellens HJJ. Dual conduction in a Mahaim fiber. *J Cardiovasc Electrophysiol* 2004;15:1212.

CHAPTER 4

The short AV decrementally conducting fibers

Decrementally conducting accessory pathways bypassing the tricuspid annulus and inserting at the anteroapical region of the right ventricle in or close to the right bundle branch have atrioventricular (AV) node-like features [1–7]. Current evidence suggests that they are an accessory conduction system with a proximal AV node-like structure and distal branching resembling the His-Purkinje system [3–8].

However, our understanding of decrementally conducting AV fibers inserting close to the tricuspid annulus is less clear. A better characterization of these fibers is hampered by their rare occurrence. The few reported series [9, 10] are small and show, apart from their decremental properties, no consistent features suggesting the presence of an accessory AV node. We carried out a retrospective study [11] to assess the electrocardiographic and electrophysiological characteristics of 8 patients with short decrementally conducting fibers and to compare these findings with a group of 33 patients with atriofascicular pathways.

Definitions

Decremental conduction A cycle length dependent prolongation of the impulse conduction time of at least 30 milliseconds through the accessory pathway.

Atriofascicular pathway: The His bundle deflection is inscribed after the right bundle deflection during maximal preexcitation. At maximal ventricular preexcitation, there was a constant QRS-His relationship without further changes from shortening the atrial pacing cycle length. Ventricular activation at the right ventricular apex occurred earlier than at the tricuspid annulus.

Short AV decrementally conducting fiber: A decrementally conducting AV pathway showing ventricular activation at the tricuspid annulus during maximal preexcitation earlier than at the right ventricular apical region (Fig. 4.1).

Also, the His bundle deflection is always inscribed before the right bundle deflection either during sinus rhythm or during atrial pacing with maximal preexcitation (Fig. 4.2).

Study population

We retrospectively studied 47 consecutive patients from four institutions having accessory pathways with long anterograde conduction times and

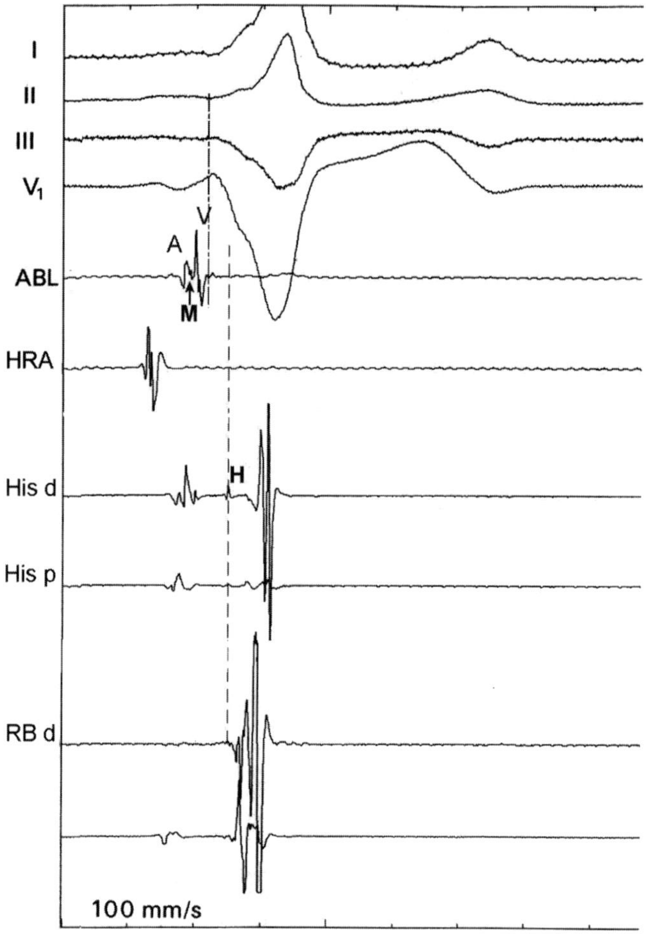

Figure 4.1 Case 2. Mapping at the lateral aspect of the tricuspid annulus shows early ventricular activation and a likely accessory pathway ("M") potential between the atrial and ventricular deflections (arrow). The ventricular activation of the right bundle branch occurs after activation at the tricuspid annulus.

decremental properties during sinus rhythm, usually suffering from a tachycardia with anterograde conduction over the decremental pathway, in whom ablation of the accessory pathway was performed. Six patients were ablated targeting the distal insertion of the atriofascicular pathway and were excluded from this study.

Every patient included in this series showed a decrementally conducting AV or atriofascicular bypass tract with progressive atrioventricular and AH interval prolongation coupled with a decreasing HV interval leading to a greater degree of ventricular preexcitation with a left bundle branch block (LBBB)-like morphology during atrial pacing [2] (Fig. 4.3).

Group A consisted of 8 patients with a short AV fiber (Fig. 4.4). There were 5 females and 3 males. Patients 1 and 2 were brothers. Their age ranged from

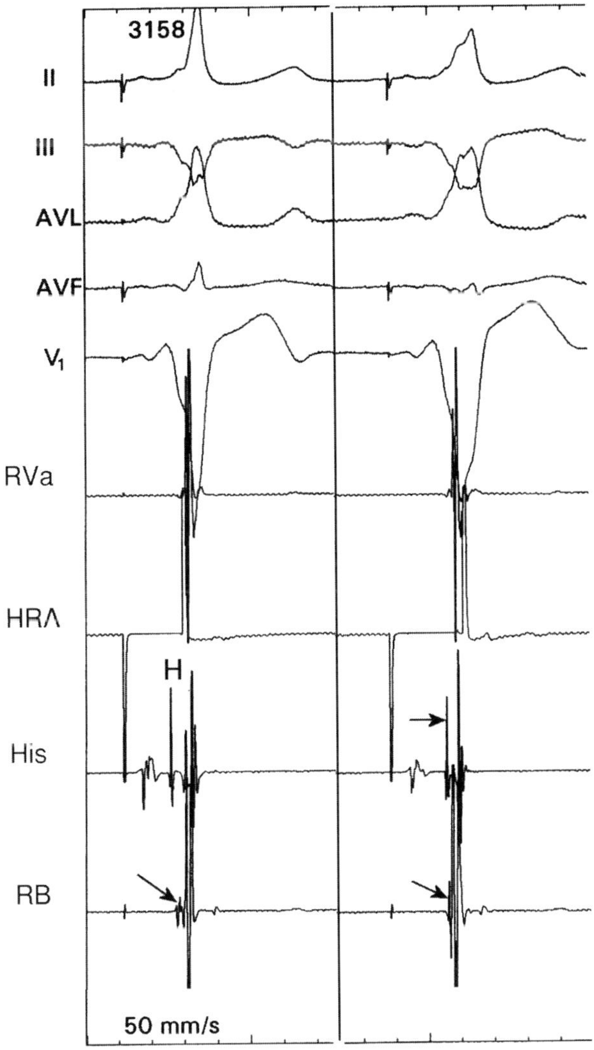

Figure 4.2 Case 2. Lack of reversal of the normal sequence of the His–right bundle branch depolarization during atrial pacing with increasing rates.

18 to 45 (mean 34 ± 8) years. One patient (case 7) had Ebstein's disease and 3 patients had an associated rapidly conducting bypass tract (Table 4.1). Four patients had recurrent tachycardias, three of them were preexcited, and one had an orthodromic AV reentrant tachycardia without bystander conduction over the short AV fiber. Only one tachycardia was related to a short AV fiber. The other three tachycardias became noninducible after ablation of their associated rapidly conducting bypass tracts. Patient 8 had intermittent preexcitation.

Group B consisted of 20 females and 13 males, with age ranging from 8 to 52 (mean 24 ± 10) years. All patients were referred for electrophysiological assessment of a wide QRS tachycardia. Preexcited AV node reentrant tachycardia

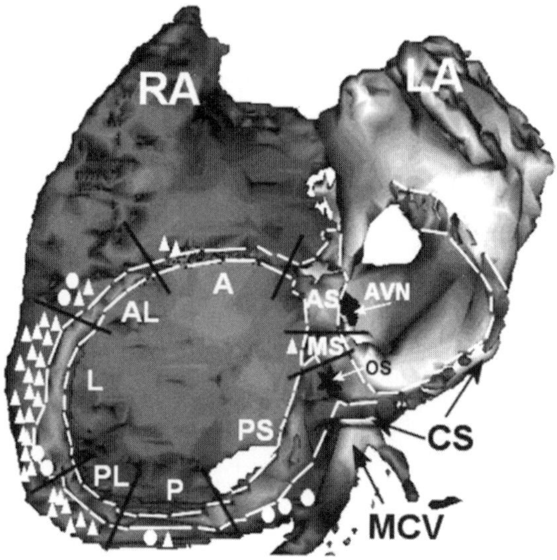

Figure 4.3 Schematic illustration showing the site of successful catheter ablation of all decremental accessory pathways in this present series in a left anterior oblique view. The tricuspid and the mitral fibrous annulus were marked for the sake of clarity. This anatomic 3-D model was built up from images obtained from the visible human project (http://visiblehuman.epfl.ch/). A, anterior; AL, anterolateral; AS, anteroseptal; AVN, AV node; CS, coronary sinus; LA, left atrium; MCV, middle cardiac vein; OS, coronary sinus ostium; P, posterior; PL, posterolateral; PS, posteroseptal; RA, right atrium. Triangles designate atriofascicular fibers; circles, short AV fibers.

using an atriofascicular pathway as a bystander was present in 1 patient. One patient had atrial fibrillation with preexcited QRS complexes, and 2 patients were referred because of repetitive episodes of unsustained tachycardia caused by automaticity arising in the atriofascicular fiber [7]. Ebstein's disease was diagnosed in 4 (12%) patients.

Adenosine test

Adenosine triphosphate was administered as a rapid intravenous bolus during atrial pacing. A bolus of 6 mg was followed by another of 12 mg when needed. A nonresponder was defined as no delay or block in AV conduction (prolonged P-delta interval or blocked P waves) in spite of the injection of up to 12 mg of adenosine.

Preablation ECG findings

Group A: All 8 patients had clear ventricular preexcitation on their baseline 12-lead ECG. In 6 patients, ventricular preexcitation occurred because of impulse conduction over a decrementally conducting short AV fiber. Two of the 8 patients showed preexcitation due to an associated rapidly conducting AV bypass tract, one right midseptal and one right anteroseptal. After ablation of these

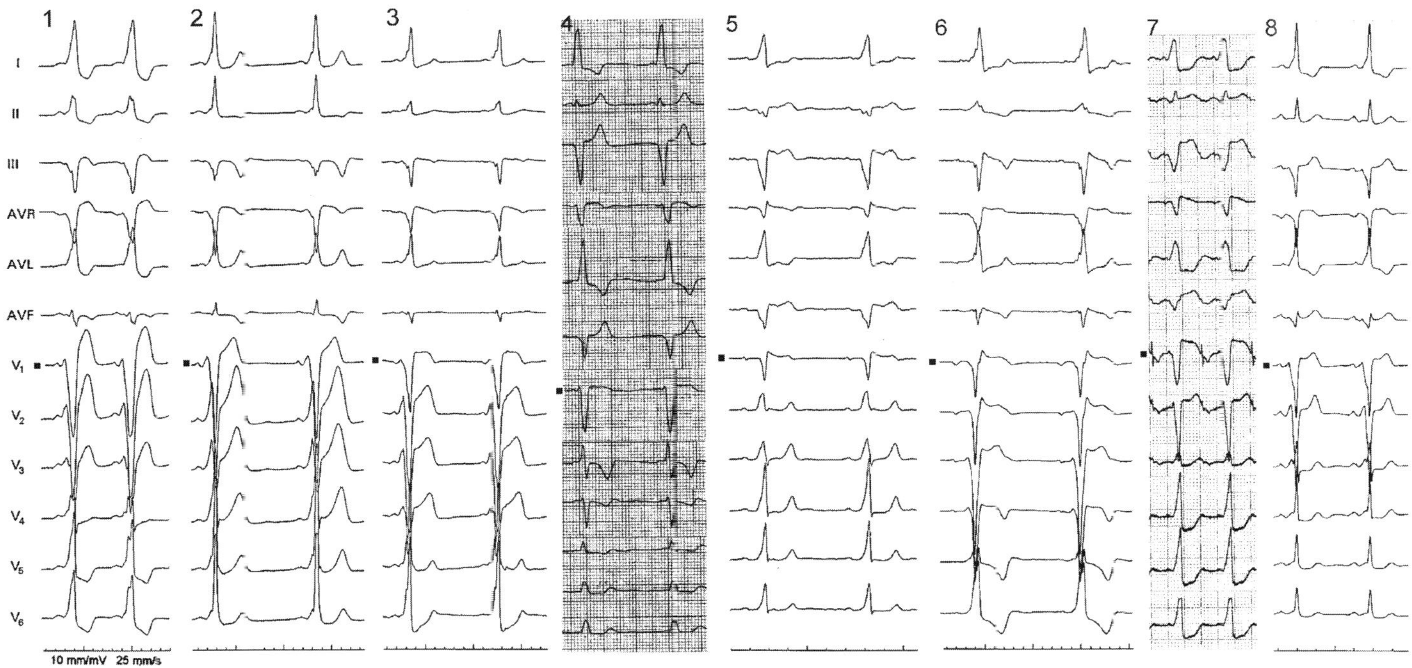

Figure 4.4 The 12-lead ECGs during anterograde conduction over a short decrementally conducting AV fiber in the 8 patients studied. Small black squares mark lead V_1. ECGs of patients 2 and 7 were recorded after ablation of an associated midseptal and right anteroseptal bypass tract respectively. Patient 7 (with Ebstein's disease) showed preexcitation only during atrial pacing (after ablation of an additional anteroseptal accessory pathway, the baseline ECG showed sinus rhythm with RBBB).

Table 4.1 Clinical, electrocardiographic, and electrophysiological data of the 8 patients with a short decrementally conducting AV fiber.

		ECG				Electrophysiological study								
Case	*Sex*	*Age*	*PR*	*QRS*	*Overt*	*AP site*	*Anti-CMT*	*M potential*	*M site*	*V-RB*	*Max dec*	*W*	*Adenosine*	*MAT*
1	M	34	0.08	0.16	yes	cRAS		no	RAL	−35	120	290		yes
2	M	36	0.08	0.16	yes	RMS		yes	RL	−60	60	300		no
3	M	41	0.08	0.17	yes			yes	RAL	−50	50	320		no
4	F	18	0.09	0.16	yes			yes	RP	−40	70	320	block	yes
5	F	40	0.14	0.16	yes			yes	RPS	−45	60	280	block	yes
6	F	45	0.16	0.18	yes		yes	no	RPS	−38	60	320	no effect	no
7	F	24	0.14	RBBB	no	RAS		yes	RPS	−40	40	430	no effect	no
8	F	34	0.12	0.16	yes			yes	RL	−40	30	700	block	yes

Abbreviations: Anti-CMT, antidromic circus movement tachycardia; AP site, bypass tract location; block, conduction block in the short AV fiber; F, female; M site, short AV fiber location; M, male; M potential, Mahaim potential; MAT, Mahaim automaticity during ablation; Max dec, maximal AV decrement at the short AV fiber during atrial pacing at increasing rates; cRAS, concealed right anteroseptal; RMS, right midseptal; RAL, right anterolateral; RP, right posterior; RPS, right posteroseptal; V-RB, V–right bundle interval during maximal preexcitation; W, Wenckebach block.

pathways, one patient (case 2) showed another preexcitation pattern due to a decrementally conducting short AV fiber and patient 7 (with Ebstein's disease) showed no preexcitation (but only RBBB) during sinus rhythm, with preexcitation becoming apparent during atrial pacing (Fig. 4.4). In the 7 patients with clear preexcitation during sinus rhythm, the PR interval was normal in 2 patients (cases 5 and 6) and short (<0.12 s) in 5 patients. As shown in Fig. 4.4, the ECG during preexcitation is similar to the ECG in patients with a rapidly conducting right-sided accessory pathway.

Group B: Five patients had an associated rapidly conducting accessory pathway. After ablation, no patient showed clear preexcitation. Twenty-four patients had a minimal preexcitation pattern, showing a QRS complex less than 0.12 seconds with an rS pattern in lead III; this was the most prevalent finding (16 of the 20 patients also showed absence of septal q waves in lead I) [12]. Two patients had an rsR′ in lead III and 2 patients had absence of septal q waves in leads I and V_6 as the only ECG clue for diagnosing minimal preexcitation [12].

Electrophysiological findings

Group A: During atrial pacing at increasing rates, mean maximal prolongation of the A-delta interval was 61 ± 26 (range 30–120) milliseconds. Wenckebach block over the short AV fiber (Fig. 4.5) occurred with a paced atrial cycle length

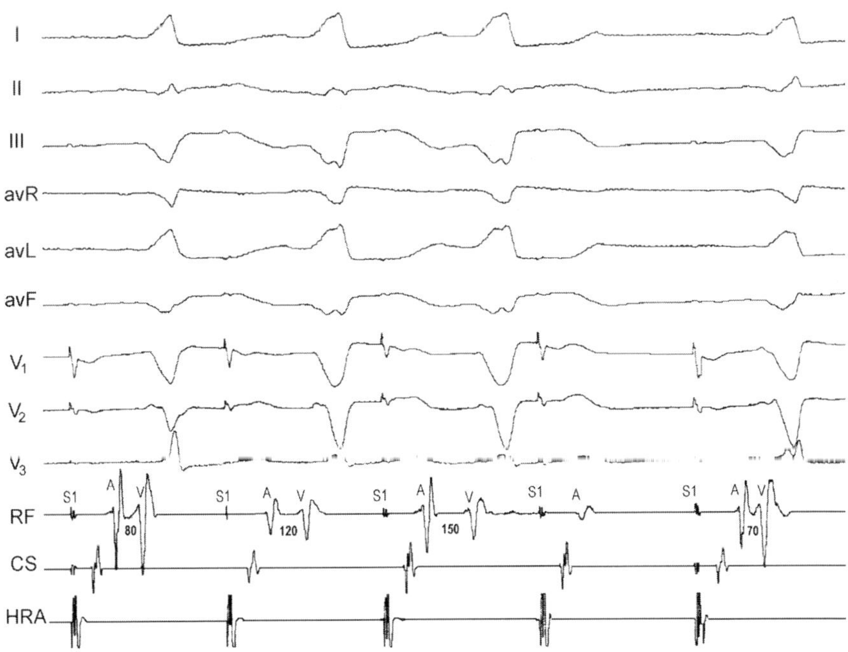

Figure 4.5 Case 7. Wenckebach block in a short AV fiber during right atrial pacing at 430 ms. The ablation catheter (RF) recorded an early ventricular electrogram at the annulus. Recording speed was 100 mm/s.

ranging from 700 to 280 milliseconds. During maximal preexcitation the mean onset QRS-RBB interval was 43 ± 8 (range 25–50) milliseconds. No patient showed reversal of His-right bundle potentials during maximal preexcitation. Only one patient (Table 4.1) had an antidromic tachycardia with anterograde conduction over the short AV fiber. Three patients had orthodromic tachycardia with their rapidly conducting AP as the retrograde limb of the circuit. None of these patients showed bystander anterograde conduction over the decremental pathway. The short decrementally conducting accessory pathways were mapped by activation mapping and ablated at an anterolateral (2 patients), lateral (2 patients), posterior (1 patient) and posteroseptal (3 patients) location. An "M" potential, which was not specifically looked for, was recorded in 6 of the 8 patients.

The M potential can be difficult to assess because it merges with the early local ventricular electrogram. In patient 8, we were able to document intermittent merging of the M potential and the local ventricular electrogram during preexcited beats, because during nonpreexcited QRS complex, spontaneous conduction block over the short AV fiber occurred in its ventricular insertion, distally to the M potential (Fig. 4.6). During radiofrequency (RF) ablation, a Mahaim automatic tachycardia occurred in 4 of the 8 patients. In 2 patients the automatic rhythm was short-lived and consisted of only three beats followed by sinus rhythm without preexcitation (Fig. 4.7).

Group B: During atrial pacing, patients with atriofascicular pathways showed Wenckebach block and maximal A-delta prolongation with no significant differences from group A patients. Mean onset QRS-RBB interval during maximal preexcitation was -6 ± 8 milliseconds ($p < 0.0001$ compared with short AV fibers). Thirty of the 33 patients had automaticity during RF catheter ablation (Table 4.2).

Adenosine test

Five patients in group A and 12 patients in group B were tested. Three of the 5 patients (60%) and 11 of the 12 patients (92%), respectively, responded with conduction block in the decrementally conducting accessory pathway (Fig. 4.8).

Common features in patients with decrementally conducting short AV fibers

The presence of overt preexcitation in 7 of the 8 patients can be explained by the large mass of right ventricular myocardium depolarized by the impulse conducted over the short fiber before the arrival of the wavefront proceeding over the His-Purkinje axis. No reversal of the His bundle–right bundle branch activation occurs because when the wavefront over the short AV fiber reaches the right bundle branch region, the His bundle and right bundle branch are already activated (Figs. 4.1 & 4.2). Maximal decremental conduction was not different between groups A and B. No patient had retrograde conduction over the anterogradely decrementally conducting fiber.

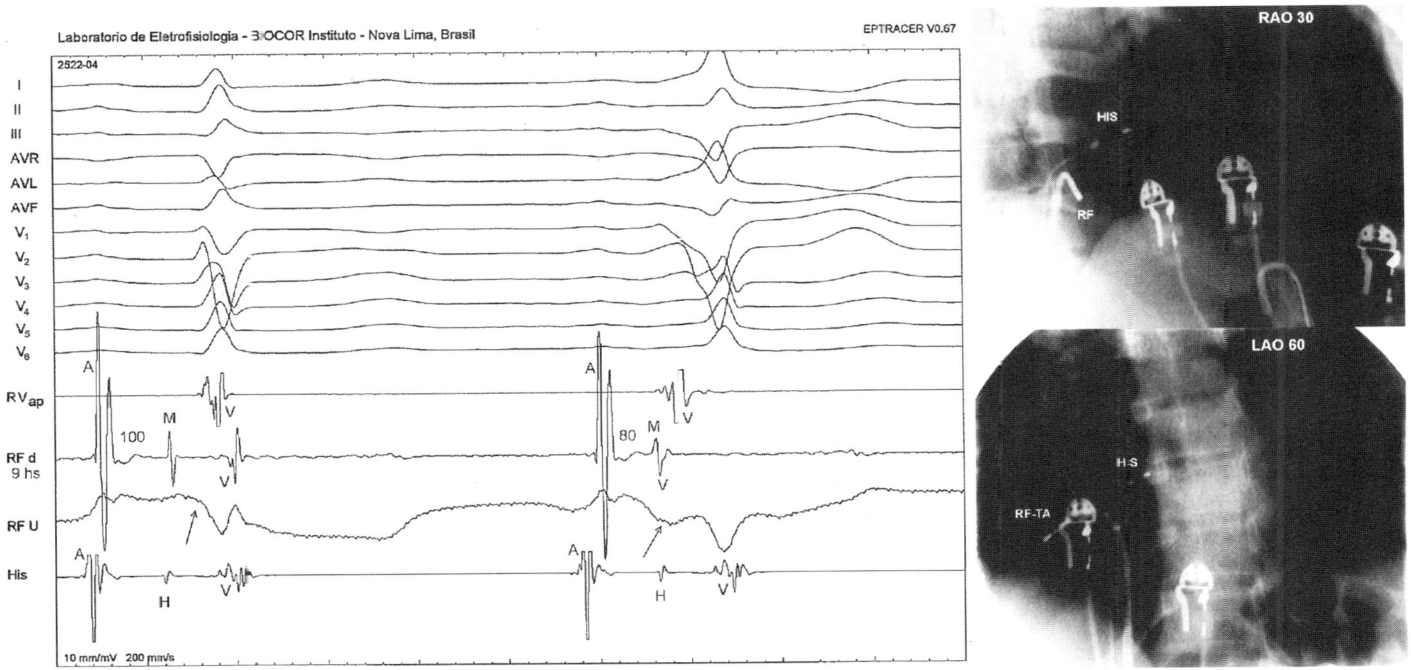

Figure 4.6 Case 8. Intermittent conduction over a short AV. The first QRS complex is not preexcited. An accessory pathway potential ("M") was recorded at the right lateral annulus. The local ventricular electrogram at the lateral aspect of the tricuspid annulus-TA (8:30 o'clock in LAO projection) is recorded after the ventricular electrogram at the apex. The next beat shows preexcitation. The local ventricular electrogram was recorded before the electrogram of the RV apex and merges with the "M" potential. The morphology of the His bundle electrogram and the AH interval does not change during the tracing. Shown are recordings from surface leads and intracardiac electrogram from the right ventricular apex (RV apex), bipolar (RF) and distal unipolar (RFu) from the ablation catheter, and His bundle (His). Recording speed is 200 mm/s. RAO (upper) and LAO fluoroscopic views of the catheters were located at the ablation site and at the bundle of His.

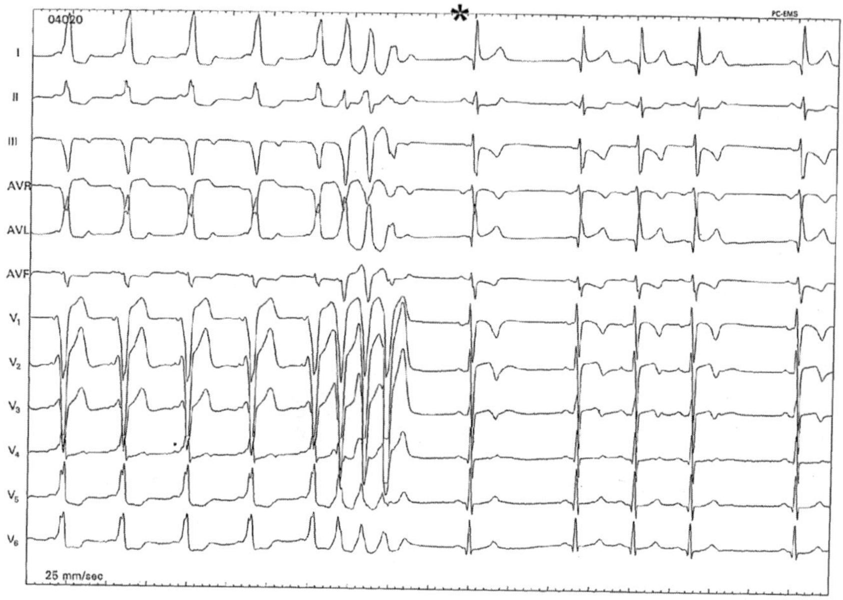

(a)

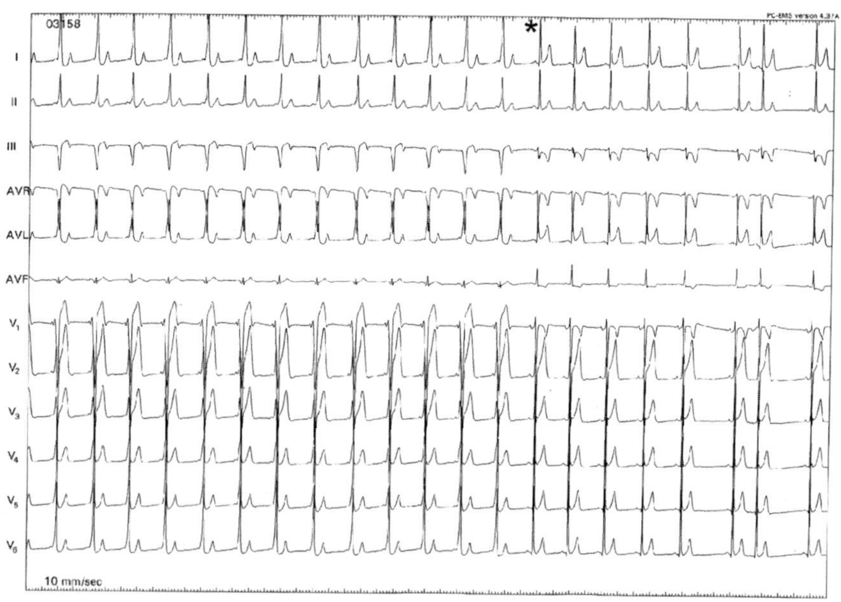

(b)

Figure 4.7 (a) Case 1. A short run of heat-induced automatic rhythm from the short AV fiber occurring just before block. (b) Case 2. Successful RFCA (*) was carried out without automatic activity.

Table 4.2 Comparative analysis between short (group A) and long (group B) decrementally conducting fibers.

Variables	*Group A*	*Group B*	p *value*
Female gender	63% (5/8)	60% (20)	ns
Mean age	34 ± 8	24 ± 10	0.02
Minimal preexcitation	0%	72% (24)	0.08
No preexcitation*	13% (1)	28% (9)	ns
Overt preexcitation*	88% (7)	0%	< 0.0001
Associated WPW	25% (2)	15% (5)	ns
Associated CBT	13% (1)	6% (2)	ns
Ebstein	13% (1)	12% (4)	ns
Antidromic CMT	13% (1)	88% (29)	ns
Block with adenosine	3/5 (60%)	11/12 (92%)	ns
M potential	75% (6)	100% (33)	ns
Mahaim automaticity	50% (4)	91% (30)	ns

*After ablation of associated bypass tracts.
CBT, concealed bypass tract; CMT, circus movement tachycardia; M, Mahaim; Mahaim automaticity, during radiofrequency ablation; ns, nonsignificant *p* value.

Discordant features in patients with decrementally conducting short AV fibers

The response to an intravenous bolus of adenosine was not uniform in group A patients. In 3 out of the 5 patients tested, conduction block developed at the AP level. Group B patients showed a different response. Adenosine induced conduction block in the atriofascicular fiber in 11 of the 12 patients tested. Other authors also found that atriofascicular pathways are sensitive to adenosine [8, 13].

Another difference was the occurrence of heat-induced automaticity during RF catheter ablation. Only 4 group A patients (50%) showed ectopic activity arising in the decrementally conducting pathway in contrast to 30 (91%) of the 33 group B patients.

AV node-like features

Patients 4, 5, and 8 responded to adenosine and had automaticity emerging during RF ablation. Patient 1 showed heat-induced automaticity but did not respond to adenosine. The electrophysiological profile of these patients did not differ from that of patients with atriofascicular pathways, who also responded to adenosine (92%) and showed accessory pathway automaticity during ablation (91%). Braun *et al.* [14] reported similar heat-induced automaticity in his 15 patients (100%) with atriofascicular pathways. We hypothesize that this subset of patients with short AV fibers who respond to adenosine and show RF-induced automaticity may have an accessory AV node without a long branching portion as found in patients with atriofascicular pathways. This substrate could be similar to the accessory node-like structure described by Becker *et al.* [15] at the lateral tricuspid valve annulus that connected to

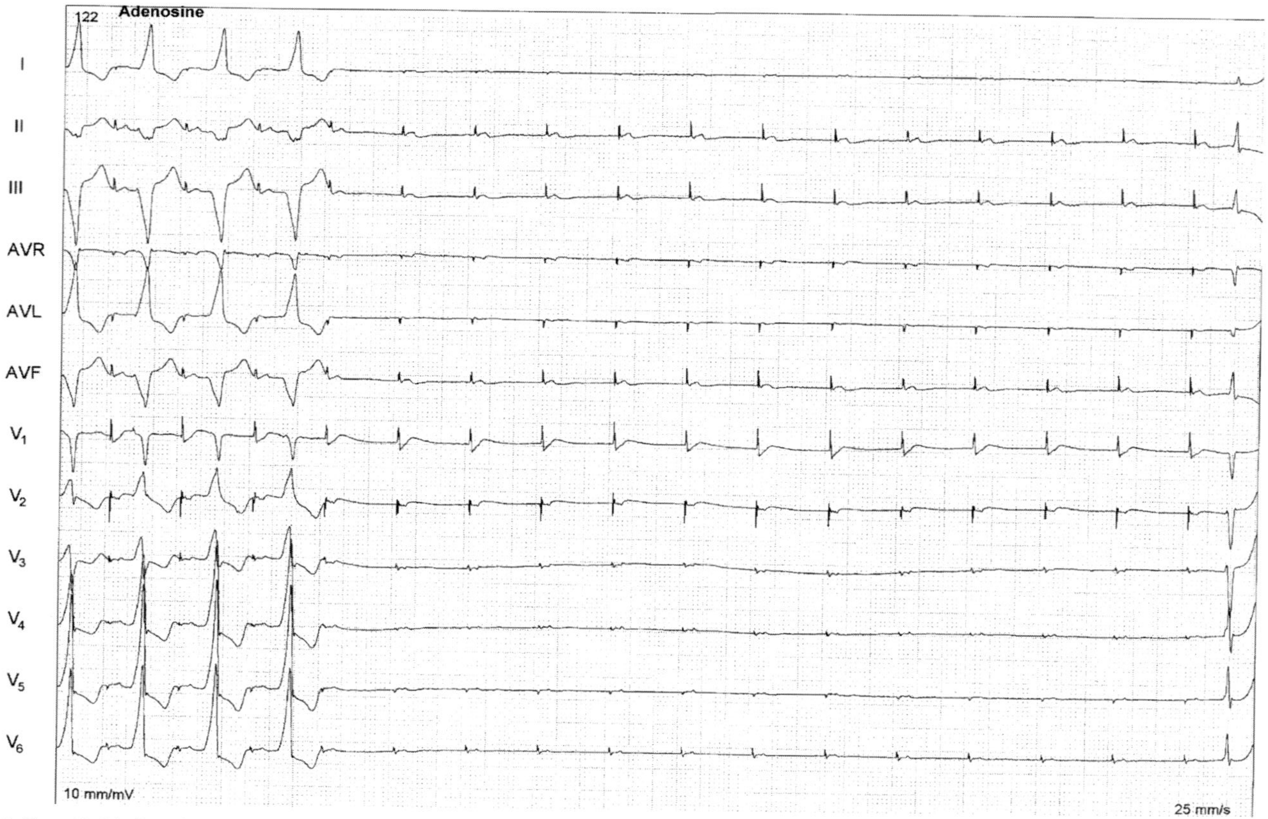

Figure 4.8 Case 5. A bolus of 6 mg of adenosine causes block of the atrial paced beats in both the AV node and the decrementally conducting short AV fiber.

the ventricular myocardium beneath the annulus in a patient with Ebstein's disease and an additional posteroseptal accessory pathway.

Decrementally conducting short AV fibers without AV node-like behavior

Patients 6 and 7 did not respond to adenosine or develop automaticity during RF ablation. Patients 2 and 3 did not have automaticity during ablation but were not given adenosine. It is still possible that patients 2 and 3 had an AV node-like structure, because not all atriofascicular patients show heat-induced automaticity.

Decremental conduction can occur for reasons other than an AV node-like structure. Haissaguerre [10] reported a patient who developed decremental conduction after an attempt of RF catheter ablation over a previous rapidly conducting accessory pathway. Critelli *et al.* [16, 17] reported one patient with the permanent form of atrioventricular reciprocating tachycardia that developed decremental anterograde conduction over a posteroseptal accessory pathway after AV node ablation. Histological examination showed no AV node-like tissue but an accessory pathway with a serpiginous course.

Do all short decrementally conducting AV fibers require catheter ablation therapy?

Only one patient in group A had a short AV fiber incorporated in a reentrant tachycardia circuit in contrast to 29 from 33 patients with atriofascicular pathways ($p = 0.09$). In addition, 2 patients had a very long effective refractory period. Patients without tachycardia and with a very long effective refractory period probably do not need ablative therapy.

Previous studies

There are very few data on decrementally conducting short AV fibers. Heald *et al.* [9] reported 4 patients with short AV fibers in a series of 21 patients with decrementally conducting accessory pathways. All 4 patients showed overt preexcitation and were ablated at the tricuspid annulus. An M potential was found in 2 of the 4 patients, and they were not challenged with adenosine. Twelve of his 21 patients had automaticity during ablation (they call it "stuttering block"), but there is no mention whether the short AV fibers also showed RF-induced automaticity. Haissaguerre *et al.* [10] also reported a series of 21 patients with decrementally conducting fibers, and four of them were classified as patients with short AV fibers, all of which were preexcited during sinus rhythm as well. Two of them (50%) were tested with adenosine and did not respond. They did not mention the occurrence of automaticity during catheter ablation. Cappato *et al.* [18] had one short AV fiber in their series of 11 patients. They found an accessory pathway potential, but there is no information regarding adenosine test or automaticity during ablation.

Limitations of the study

There are some limiting factors in our study, such as the small number of patients challenged with adenosine. Our assumption of defining the group A patients as having a decrementally conducting "short AV fiber" is not based on histological data. However, there is sound electrophysiological evidence derived from local ventricular activation mapping that supports our working definition.

Conclusion

Short decrementally conducting right-sided accessory pathways show a typical ECG pattern different from that of atriofascicular pathways. However, their electrophysiological properties may not be uniform. These pathways can be successfully interrupted by catheter ablation.

References

1 Mahaim I, Bennett A. Nouvelle recherches sur les connexions supérieures de la branche gauche du faisceau de His-Tawara avec cloison interventriculaire. *Cardiologia* 1938;1:61.

2 Wellens HJJ. *Electrical Stimulation of the Heart in the Study and Treatment of Tachycardias.* Baltimore: University Park Press; 1971.

3 Klein GJ, Guiraudon GM, Kerr CR, *et al.* "Nodoventricular" accessory pathway: evidence for a distinct accessory atrioventricular pathway with atrioventricular node-like properties. *J Am Coll Cardiol* 1988;11:1035.

4 Guiraudon CM, Guiraudon GM, Klein GJ. Histologic evidence for an accessory atrioventricular pathway with AV-node-like morphology. *Circulation* 1988;78(suppl 2):40.

5 Ellenbogen KA, Ramirez NM, Packer DL, *et al.* Accessory nodoventricular (Mahaim) fibers. A clinical review. *Pacing Clin Electrophysiol* 1986;9:868.

6 Sternick EB, Gerken LM, Vrandecic MO. Appraisal of "Mahaim" automatic tachycardia. *J Cardiovasc Electrophysiol* 2002;13:244.

7 Sternick EB, Sosa EA, Timmermans C, *et al.* Automaticity in Mahaim fibers. *J Cardiovasc Electrophysiol* 2004;15:738.

8 McClelland JH, Wang X, Beckman KJ, *et al.* Radiofrequency catheter ablation of right atriofascicular (Mahaim) accessory pathways guided by accessory pathway activation potentials. *Circulation* 1994;89:2655.

9 Heald SC, Davies DW, Ward DE, *et al.* Radiofrequency catheter ablation of Mahaim tachycardia by targeting Mahaim potentials at the tricuspid annulus. *Br Heart J* 1995;73:250.

10 Haissaguerre M, Cauchemez B, Marcus F, *et al.* Characteristics of the ventricular insertion sites of accessory pathways with anterograde decremental conduction properties. *Circulation* 1995;91:1077.

11 Sternick EB, Fagundes M, Cruz Filho FE, *et al.* Short atrioventricular Mahaim fiber: observations on their clinical, eletrocardiographic and electrophysiologic profile. *J Cardiovasc Electrophysiol* 2005;16:127.

12 Sternick EB, Timmermans C, Sosa EA, *et al.* The electrocardiogram in sinus rhythm and tachycardia in patients with Mahaim fibers. The importance of an "rS" pattern in lead III. *J Am Coll Cardiol* 2004;44:1626.

13 Ellenbogen KA, Rogers R, Old W. Pharmacological characterization of conduction over a Mahaim fiber: evidence for adenosine sensitive conduction. *Pacing Clin Electrophysiol* 1989;12:1396.

14 Braun E, Siebbels J, Volkmer M, *et al.* Radiofrequency-induced preexcited automatic rhythm during ablation accessory pathways with Mahaim-type preexcitation: does it predict clinical outcome? *Pacing Clin Electrophysiol* 1997;20:1121.

15 Becker AE, Anderson RH, Durrer D, Wellens HJJ. The anatomical substrates of Wolff–Parkinson–White syndrome: a clinicopathologic correlation in seven patients. *Am J Cardiol* 1981;48:47.

16 Critelli G, Perticone F, Coltorti F, *et al.* Antegrade slow bypass conduction after closed-chest ablation of the His bundle in permanent junctional reciprocating tachycardia. *Circulation* 1983;67:687.

17 Critelli G, Gallagher JJ, Monda V, *et al.* Anatomic and electrophysiologic substrate of the permanent form of junctional reciprocating tachycardia. *J Am Coll Cardiol* 1984;4:601.

18 Cappato R, Schluter M, Weiss C, *et al.* Catheter-induced mechanical conduction block of right sided accessory fibers with Mahaim-type preexcitation to guide radiofrequency ablation. *Circulation* 1994;90:282.

CHAPTER 5

Nodoventricular and Nodofascicular fibers

Nodoventricular (NV) and nodofascicular (NF) fibers together with the fasciculoventricular pathway (discussed in chapter 7) comprise the "genuine" Mahaim fibers, as originally described by Dr Ivan Mahaim in his historic manuscript [1], published in the late 1930s. Since the 1980s, when it became clear that the majority of the fibers that were previously called nodoventricular were in reality atriofascicular pathways, some authors even doubted the very existence of such structures. In the last 25 years we have learned that NV and NF fibers do exist, but only a few well-studied cases have been reported [2–17].

The hallmark electrocardiographic feature of a tachycardia using an NV or an NF fiber either as the anterograde or retrograde limb of a macro-reentry circuit is atrioventricular (AV) dissociation, because the atria are not part of the circuit. Gallagher *et al.* [5] reported three patients with ventriculoatrial (VA) dissociation, but detailed tracings were shown for only one patient with Ebstein's disease, a Klippel–Feil syndrome, and an atrial septal defect (ASD). This patient had an left bundle branch block (LBBB)-like tachycardia with 2:1 VA conduction and another tachycardia with RBBB and a normal HV interval also showing 2:1 VA block, considered by the authors to represent the reversed circuit. As we will discuss, the major differential diagnosis of a tachycardia incorporating an NV/NF fiber is ventricular tachycardia, in case of a wide QRS complex tachycardia, and AV nodal reentry tachycardia (AVNRT) with VA block; intrahisian reentry in patients with a narrow, complex QRS tachycardia; intraventricular reentry high in the septum; interfascicular reentrant tachycardia; and junctional ectopic tachycardia (JET).

Electrophysiology

Figure 5.1 shows the varieties of fibers taking off from the AV node that have been reported. The tachycardia can be antidromic, with VA conduction or AV dissociation, or orthodromic, typically with AV dissociation (Fig. 5.2).

Proof of the participation of the NV/NF fiber in the tachycardia circuit

Proof that the NF fiber is part of the orthodromic circuit is provided by advancement of the next His bundle potential by a ventricular premature beat

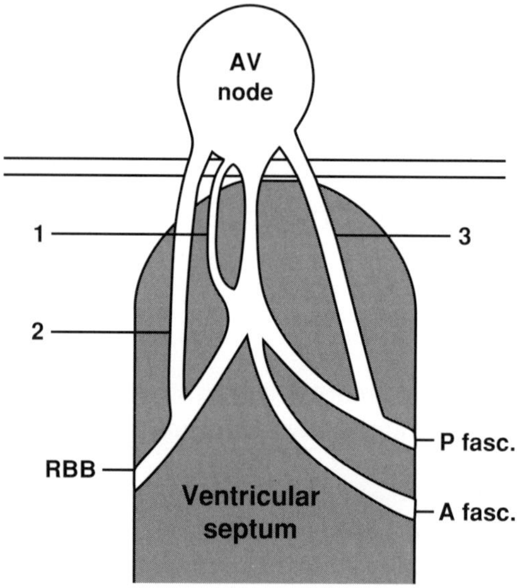

Figure 5.1 Varieties of Mahaim fibers with a proximal insertion at the AV node: 1, a nodo-His fiber [12]; 2, NV or NF fibers [5, 8, 11, 14]; 3, a left-sided NV or NF fiber connected with the posterior fascicle of the left bundle, as reported by Okishige and Friedman [13].

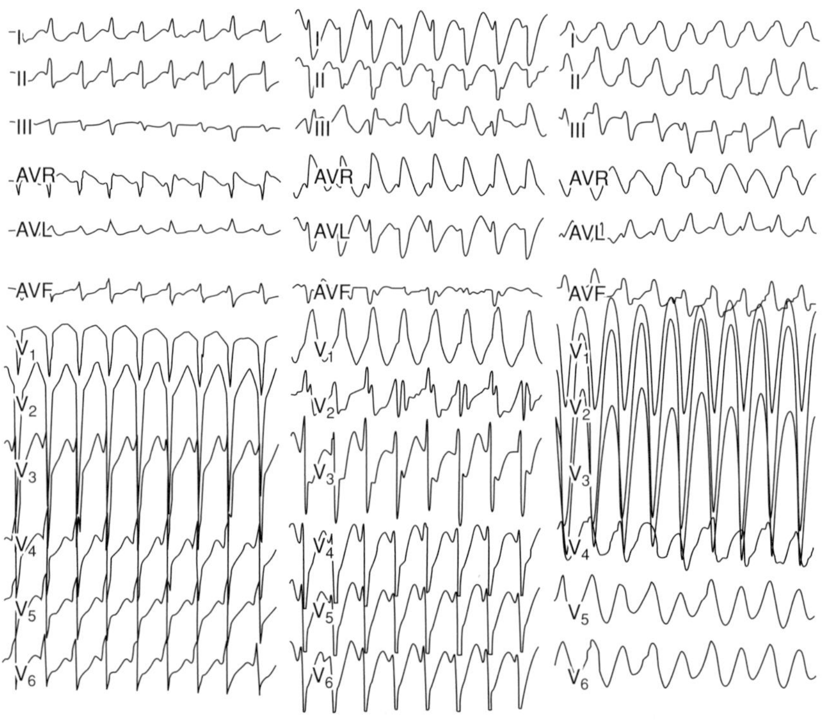

Figure 5.2 A patient with a concealed NF fiber: 12-lead ECGs during narrow QRS tachycardia, tachycardia with RBBB pattern, and tachycardia with a LBBB without change in the tachycardia cycle length. During narrow QRS complex tachycardia, AV dissociation is best seen in lead II. QRS alternans is most outspoken in leads III and AVL. Courtesy of Haissaguerre *et al.* [12].

delivered during His bundle refractoriness. Such a maneuver can also be used to identify the distal end of the pathway.

On the other hand, failure to advance ventricular activity by a late atrial premature stimulus delivered during antidromic tachycardia does not necessarily imply the presence of an NV pathway, as pointed out by Porkolab *et al.* [18]. Definite proof that an atriofascicular pathway was present was achieved by effective radiofrequency (RF) catheter ablation in the right lateral groove, guided by an "M" potential.

Definition of the fiber insertion sites

Distal end: In patients with an NF or NV fiber having anterograde conduction, the distal insertion site can be assessed by doing activation mapping. NF fibers would show, as in atriofascicular pathways, the earliest activation at the apex and late activation at the annulus. However, in patients having a concealed NF fiber, assessment of the distal end can be achieved by delivering, at the time of His bundle refractoriness, premature ventricular extrastimulus during tachycardia at different ventricular sites, looking for the greatest amount of HH shortening.

Another helpful maneuver is to assess the tachycardia cycle length during narrow QRS complex and during transient right and left bundle branch block. When the tachycardia cycle length does not change with bundle branch block, the lower turnaround of the circuit should be located above the His bundle bifurcation (Fig. 5.2). Also, the occurrence of a transient 2:1 infrahisian AV block is consistent with a fiber being connected to the His bundle or the upper part of the right bundle branch.

Proximal end: When complete AV dissociation occurs during tachycardia, it is clear that the proximal insertion site should be located in the distal part of the AV node. In the case of a patient showing 1:1 VA conduction and transient 2:1 infrahisian AV block, an atrial tachycardia can be excluded by tachycardia termination with a premature ventricular extrastimulus delivered during His bundle refractoriness. The observation of alternation of the AH interval during tachycardia is consistent with a connection to the proximal part of the AV node. The least elegant maneuver is to attempt RF catheter ablation at the proximal end, as described by Okishige and Friedman [13]. They reported complete AV nodal block and ablation of an NV fiber with the application of a single pulse of radiofrequency at a midseptal site.

Retrograde VH conduction

In spite of the absence of a direct VA connection, some patients may have retrograde decremental VH conduction. Reversal of the depolarization sequence of the His and the right bundle branch potentials was observed by Haissaguerre *et al.* [12]. During ventricular pacing, the right bundle branch potential preceded the recording of the His bundle potential. However, at a critical cycle

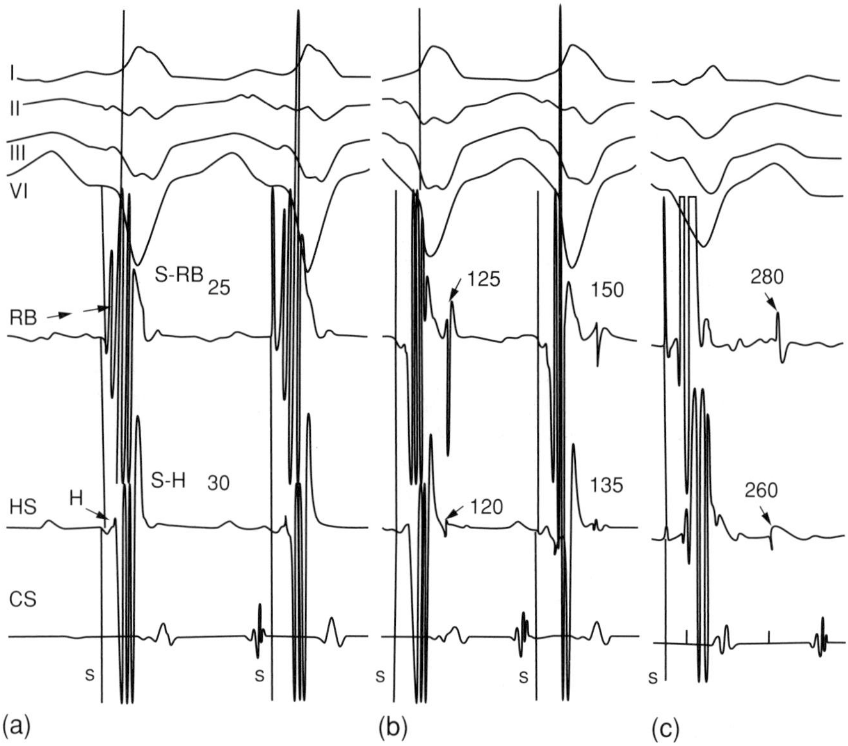

Figure 5.3 Retrograde conduction sequences during right ventricular pacing. The values given indicate the intervals between pacing spike(s) and right bundle branch and His electrograms. Ventricular pacing at a cycle length of 420 ms (a) depolarizes the proximal RB first and then the His bundle 5 ms later. At a pacing cycle length of 330 ms (b), the His bundle becomes activated before the right bundle, and this activation sequence remains the same at increasing ventricular pacing rates. At a short pacing cycle length (c), there is a long conduction time of 260 ms to the His bundle. Note that the atrial electrogram has no relation to ventricular activation (bottom lead). CS, coronary sinus. Courtesy of Haissaguerre *et al.* [12].

length, there was a VH jump, with the His bundle potential now being recorded before the right bundle potential (Fig. 5.3). This could be explained by conduction block at the right bundle branch, proximal to the NF insertion site with retrograde conduction over the NF fiber and anterograde conduction over the His bundle. However, transseptal conduction followed by retrograde conduction over the left bundle branch could also explain these findings.

Differential diagnosis

The differential diagnosis of a regular tachycardia, with a narrow QRS complex and AV dissociation (V > A) includes the following: (i) orthodromic reentrant tachycardia using an NF or NV pathway as the retrograde limb; (ii) AVNRT with VA block [2, 19, 20]; (iii) His bundle tachycardia with VA block [21]; (iv) interfascicular reentrant tachycardia; and (v) junctional ectopic tachycardia (JET).

An AVNRT with HA block is unlikely when a ventricular premature extrastimulus delivered during tachycardia at the time of His bundle refractoriness advances the HH interval. The differential diagnosis between an AVNRT and a tachycardia using a concealed NF fiber can be difficult [19]. Factors that favor a NF fiber include the following: (i) intermittent anterograde preexcitation [8]; (ii) absence of His bundle activation when the tachycardia is initiated by ventricular extrastimuli [20]; (iii) tachycardia initiation with a single atrial premature beat producing a dual ventricular response, 1:2 AV conduction [20]; (iv) increase in the tachycardia cycle length at the occurrence of bundle branch block [9]; (v) ability of a ventricular extrastimulus during His bundle refractoriness to advance the next His bundle activation [12]; (vi) reproducible termination with adenosine supports participation of the AV node as the anterograde limb in the tachycardia circuit; and (vii) catheter ablation of the AV node or the NV fiber with elimination of the tachycardia.

Intrahisian reentry may occur in a diseased His bundle, with prolongation of the HV interval and the occurrence of a split His potential. It should not be responsive to adenosine, and a ventricular premature extrastimulus delivered during His bundle refractoriness should not reset or terminate it.

RF catheter ablation

RF ablation aimed at either a concealed NF or a manifest NV fiber carries a high risk of AV block. Okishige and Friedman [13] ablated the lower right midseptal region and observed a simultaneous block in the Mahaim fiber and the AV node. The patient needed a permanent pacemaker. Some authors, however, were successful in ablating such structures without harming the AV node His–Purkinje system. Grogin *et al.* [11] successfully ablated two NV fibers at the right midseptal region. In none of the patients, an accessory pathway – M potential – could be found. In one patient a slow AV nodal pathway was ablated in addition to the NV fiber. Haissaguerre *et al.* [12] successfully ablated a nodo-His fiber by positioning the ablation catheter beneath the tricuspid valve, at a site with a clear His bundle potential and a very low voltage atrial deflection (Fig. 5.4). Hluchy *et al.* [15] ablated a concealed NF fiber at the right midseptal region, where an AP potential was found during tachycardia. However, none of the authors mention whether junctional automaticity occurred during current delivery at the right midseptal region. Others, like Kottkamp *et al.* [14], did not need to ablate the fiber, which had a bystander role, and ablation of the slow AV nodal pathway was all that was needed to make the patient asymptomatic.

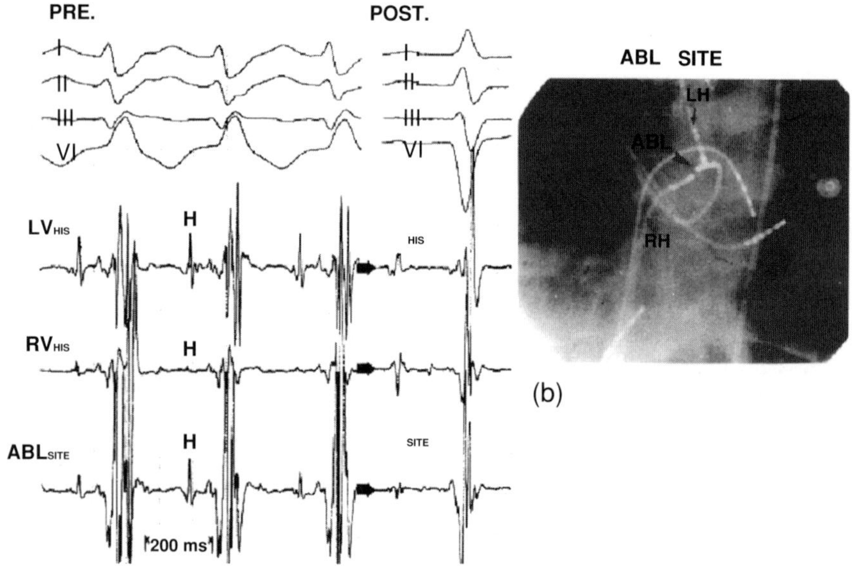

(a)

Figure 5.4 (a) Electrograms recorded from the three sites during tachycardia before ablation (pre) and during sinus rhythm after ablation (post). Note the amplitude of the His potential at the ablation site before ablation and its absence immediately after ablation with a low amplitude of the local atrial activity. The His bundle recording from the left side has also disappeared despite the fact that the catheter position was unchanged. Complete right bundle block developed a few seconds after ablation. (b) Successful ablation site as seen on the AP radiogram relative to the His bundle sites recorded from the right side (RH) or the left side (LH) of the septum. ABL, ablation catheter. Courtesy of Haissaguerre *et al*. [12].

References

1 Mahaim I, Winston MR. Recherches d'anatomie comparée et de pathologie expérimentale sur les connexions hautes du faisceau de His-Tawara. *Cardiologia* 1941;5:189.

2 Wellens HJJ. Unusual examples of reentrant supraventricular tachycardia. *Circulation* 1975;15:997.

3 Donzeau JP, Constans R, Bernardet P, *et al*. Tachycardie jonctionnelle avec dissociation auriculo-ventriculaire probablement liée à un faisceau de Mahaim inapparent en rythme sinusal. *Ann Cardiol Angéiol* 1977;26:413.

4 Saulnier JP, Nouviaire R, Aliot E, Mariot J, *et al*. Reentry tachycardia with complete atrioventricular dissociation probably connected with the right Mahaim bundle. *Arch Mal Coeur Vaiss* 1979;72:1259.

5 Gallagher JJ, Smith WM, Kassell JH, *et al*. Role of Mahaim fibers in cardiac arrhythmias in man. *Circulation* 1981;64:176.

6 Morady F, Scheinman MM, Gonzales R, *et al*. His-ventricular dissociation in a patient with reciprocating tachycardia and a nodoventricular bypass tract. *Circulation* 1981;64:839.

7 Ko PT, Naccarelli GV, Gulamhusein S, *et al*. Atrioventricular dissociation during paroxysmal junctional tachycardia. *Pacing Clin Electrophysiol* 1981;4:670.

8 Gmeiner R, Ng CK, Hammer I, Becker AE. Tachycardia caused by an accessory nodoventricular tract: a clinico-pathologic correlation. *Eur Heart J* 1984;5:233.
9 Shimizu A, Ohe T, Takaki H, *et al.* Narrow QRS complex tachycardia with atrioventricular dissociation. *Pacing Clin Electrophysiol* 1988;11:384.
10 Wu D, Yeh SJ, Yamamoto T, *et al.* Participation of a concealed nodoventricular fiber in the genesis of paroxysmal tachycardias. *Am Heart J* 1990;119:583.
11 Grogin HR, Lee RJ, Kwasman M, Epstein LM, *et al.* Radiofrequency catheter ablation of atriofascicular and nodoventricular Mahaim tracts. *Circulation* 1994;90:272.
12 Haissaguerre M, Campos J, Marcus FI, *et al.* Involvement of a nodofascicular connection in supraventricular tachycardia with VA dissociation. *J Cardiovasc Electrophysiol* 1994;5:854.
13 Okishige K, Friedman PL. New observations on decremental atriofascicular and nodoventricular fibers: implications for catheter ablation. *Pacing Clin Electrophysiol* 1995;18:986.
14 Kottkamp H, Hindricks G, Shenasa H, *et al.* Variants of preexcitation-specialized atriofascicular pathways, nodofascicular pathways, and fasciculoventricular pathways: electrophysiologic findings and target sites for radiofrequency catheter ablation. *J Cardiovasc Electrophysiol* 1996;7:916.
15 Hluchy J, Schickel S, Jörger U, *et al.* Electrophysiologic characteristics and radiofrequency ablation of concealed nodofascicular and left anterograde atriofascicular pathways. *J Cardiovasc Electrophysiol* 2000;11:211.
16 Mantovan R, Verlato R, Corrado D, *et al.* Orthodromic tachycardia with atrioventricular dissociation: evidence for a nodoventricular (Mahaim) fiber. *Pacing Clin Electrophysiol* 2000;23:276.
17 Gula LJ, Posan E, Skanes AC, *et al.* Tachycardia with VA Dissociation: an unusual mechanism. *J Cardiovasc Electrophysiol* 2005;16:663.
18 Porkolab F, Alpert B, Scheinman MM. Failure of atrial premature beats to reset atriofascicular tachycardia. *Pacing Clin Electrophysiol* 1999;22:528.
19 Calò L, Lamberti F, Ciolli A, Santini M. Atrioventricular nodal reentrant tachycardia with ventriculoatrial block and unsuccessful ablation of the slow pathway. *J Cardiovasc Electrophysiol* 2002;13:705.
20 Hamdan MH, Kalman JM, Lesh MD, *et al.* Narrow complex tachycardia with V-A block: diagnostic and therapeutic implications. *Pacing Clin Electrophysiol* 1998;21:1196.
21 Narula OS. Longitudinal dissociation in His bundle: bundle branch block due to asynchronous conduction within the His bundle in man. *Circulation* 1977;56:996.

CHAPTER 6

Fasciculoventricular fibers

Introduction

Both fasciculoventricular (FV) and nodoventricular (NV) pathways are varieties of true Mahaim fibers [1, 2]. The FV pathway is a rare variant [3–5] of preexcitation taking off from the bundle of His or the bundle branches and inserting into the ventricular septum [6]. Since Gallagher *et al.* [7] published the largest series of FV pathways (6 patients) in 1981, few additional cases were reported [8–1]. A number of reasons account for the paucity of publications, such as the rarity and underdiagnosis of FV pathway either because no cardiac arrhythmias occur or because of the small amount of ventricular preexcitation on the electrocardiogram. According to Josephson [3] it should be regarded as an electrocardiographic curiosity. Although playing no active role in tachycardia circuits, FV pathways are frequently associated with rapidly conducting bypass tracts, and in this era of therapeutic cardiac electrophysiology, one should be able to differentiate an anteroseptal para-Hisian bypass tract from a FV pathway, in particular in patients presenting with a tachycardia using an associated atrioventricular (AV) bypass tracts, to avoid harm to AV nodal conduction if they are targeted for catheter ablation [4].

Electrocardiographic recognition

The electrocardiographic (ECG) recognition of an FV pathway is based on the finding of a minimal preexcitation pattern with a normal QRS frontal plane axis with a variable PR interval [3, 7]. There are very few published data on the electrocardiogram of FV pathways [4, 5, 7, 11–13], and so we carried out a study to assess the ECG profile in a cohort of 7 patients with FV pathways and compared their characteristics with the ECG pattern of patients having AV bypass tracts inserting in the anteroseptal and midseptal region.

Differentiating FV fibers from septal bypass tracts

Study population: FV pathways (group I)

During the past 9 years, 8 patients with FV pathways (Fig. 6.1) were diagnosed out of 392 patients with manifest ventricular preexcitation who were referred to the Biocor institute for electrophysiological evaluation [5]. In 3 of the 8 patients (38%) the FV pathway could only be diagnosed after catheter ablation of a rapidly conducting bypass tract. One of the 8 patients lacked some

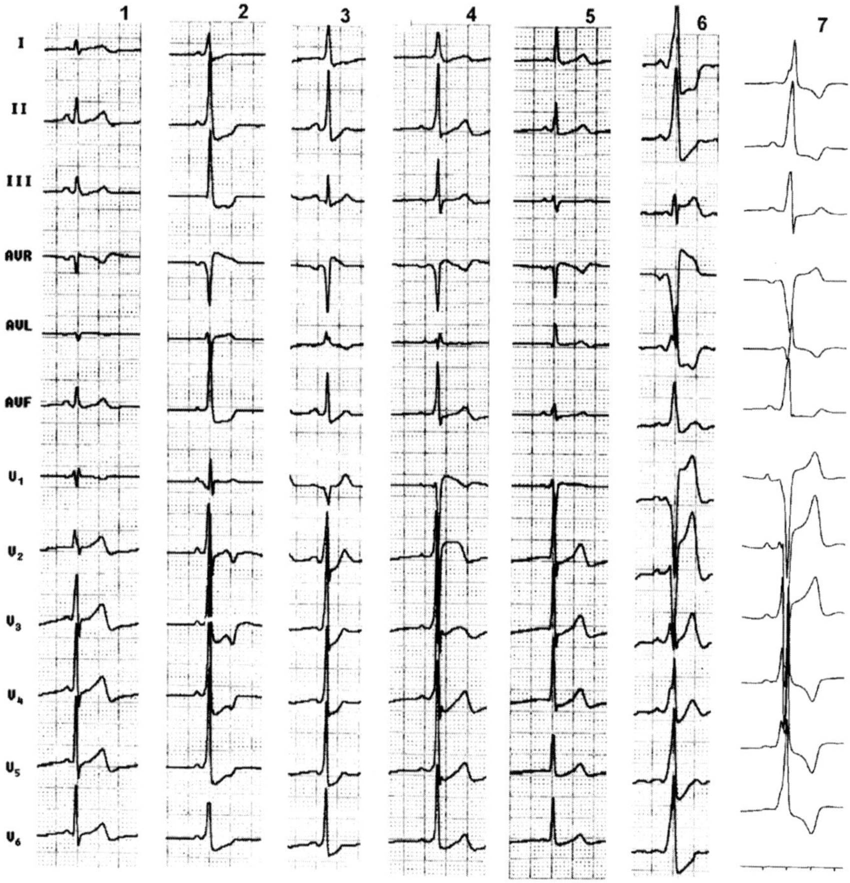

Figure 6.1 The 12-lead ECGs of 7 patients with a fasciculoventricular pathway diagnosed by an EP study. There is a wide range of presentation, ranging from a near normal QRS complex [5] to a fully preexcited QRS complex [6, 7].

electrophysiological data and was not included in this study. Another (case 3) had two rapidly conducting accessory pathways and had had an episode of aborted sudden cardiac death. Six patients were male. Their mean age was 29 ± 16 (range 13–54) years. Four patients were referred because of paroxysmal tachycardia, two were asymptomatic and were studied for risk assessment of preexcitation, and one had palpitations. Two patients (29%) had paroxysmal AV nodal reentry tachycardia (AVNRT), and one of them also had nonsustained repetitive atrial tachycardia (Table 6.1).

Group with antero- or midseptal AV accessory pathways

The group consisted of 40 patients (17 were male) with a single accessory AV pathway and a mean age of 28 ± 13 (range 12–55) years. Twenty patients had

Table 6.1 Clinical, electrocardiographic, and electrophysiological data of patients with fasciculoventricular pathways.

Case	*Age*	*Sex*	*Symptom*	*EPS*	*BT site*	*PR*	*QRS width (s)*	*QRS axis*	*Angle QRS/Delta axis*	*AH*	*HV*	*PW*
1	51	M	no			0.10	0.10	80	20	60	25	320
2	19	M	palpitations			0.09	0.12	70	40	50	25	380
3	19	M	tachycardia	WPW	LL + RMS	0.12	0.12	50	20	75	25	290
4	21	M	no			0.11	0.12	60	0	80	19	350
5	54	M	tachycardia	AVNRT		0.09	0.09	15	45	55	29	360
6	13	M	tachycardia	WPW	LL	0.11	0.15	30	30	60	20	320
7	27	F	tachycardia	AVNRT + AT		0.11	0.15	45	15	60	28	250

Angle QRS/Delta axis, difference between the frontal plane axis of QRS complex and delta wave; AT, atrial tachycardia; AVNRT, AV node reentrant tachycardia; BT, bypass tract; EPS, electrophysiological study; LL, left lateral AP; PW, Wenckebach point; QRS axis, frontal plane axis; RAS, right anteroseptal AP; RMS, right midseptal AP; WPW = Wolff-Parkinson-White syndrome.

Table 6.2 Comparative electrocardiographic findings in midseptal, anteroseptal accessory pathways and fasciculoventricular pathways.

	MS	*AS*	*FVP*	p *value*
âQRS	NA	NA	NA	
âDELTA	NA	NA	NA	
Angle between QRS and Delta wave axis	$23 \pm 8^\circ$	$4 \pm 8^\circ$	$24 \pm 15^\circ$	<0.0001 (AS vs FVP)
R/S ratio in lead III	<1 or 1	>1	<1 or >1	
2 inferior leads with a negative delta wave	0	0	0	
1 inferior leads with a negative delta wave	25%	0%	0%	
Precordial lead transition to R/S ratio > 1	$V_2 - V_3 - V_4$	$V_3 - V_4$	$V_2 - V_3 - V_4$	
QRS width	0.14 ± 0.008	0.14 ± 0.01	0.12 ± 0.02	<0.0001

âQRS, QRS frontal plane axis; âDELTA, frontal plane axis of the delta wave; AS, anteroseptal bypass tract; FVP, fasciculoventricular pathway; MS, right midseptal bypass tract; NA, normal axis; ns = not significant. Characters in bold show a higher prevalence of one value over the other.

a midseptal AP (group II) – 13 of them located close to the CS ostium and 7 located at the apical region of the triangle of Koch – and 20 patients had an anteroseptal AP (group III). We used the method described Rodriguez *et al.* [14] to analyze the electrocardiograms of patients with septal bypass tracts.

None of our patients had additional congenital or acquired cardiac abnormalities that could have affected the QRS morphology. The electrocardiograms were analyzed independently by the four authors [5]. The electrocardiographic data analyzed were as follows: QRS axis and delta wave axis in the frontal plane, the angle between the QRS and the delta wave frontal plane axis, the R/S ratio in lead III, presence of initial negativity in the inferior leads, the R/S > 1 transition in the precordial leads, the PR interval, and the QRS width (Table 6.2).

Definitions

Fasciculoventricular pathway: The baseline HV (H-delta) interval during sinus rhythm is <35 ms. During atrial pacing at increasing rates the HV interval does not change. Atrial premature beats cause progressive prolongation of the AH interval without any change in the HV interval and QRS configuration, unless block occurs in the FV pathway resulting in a normal HV interval and a narrow QRS complex. Response to adenosine triphosphate suggests an FV pathway when prolongation of the PR interval (AH interval) does not change the degree of preexcitation or complete AV block occurs after the P wave.

Anteroseptal accessory pathways (AP): These are bypass tracts lying in close proximity to or immediately anterior to the His bundle. The so-called para-Hisian bypass tracts were included in this group.

Midseptal accessory pathways: These are bypass tracts located in an area anterior to the coronary sinus and below the His bundle.

Accessory pathway location: It was established by endocardial activation mapping during sinus rhythm and validated by successful catheter ablation.

Polarity of the delta wave: The first 40-ms vector of the QRS complex.

All patients underwent an electrophysiological study after discontinuation of antiarrhythmic drug for at least 7 days (no patient was taking amiodarone).

Statistical analysis

Comparison between the accessory pathway location groups and their ECG parameters were analyzed using the two-way analysis of variance and the Student Newman–Keuls test. The values are given as mean ± standard deviation. Statistical significance was assumed for p values of <0.05.

Results

Group I (FV pathways)

After ablating all associated bypass tracts, we found the following ECG and electrophysiological findings.

Electrocardiogram during sinus rhythm (Table 6.2)

The mean PR interval was 0.10 ± 0.01 s (range 0.09–0.12). The mean QRS complex width was 0.12 ± 0.02 s (range 0.09–0.15). The QRS frontal plane axis ranged from $+15^\circ$ to $+80^\circ$ ($50^\circ \pm 22^\circ$). The mean delta wave axis in the frontal plane was $47^\circ \pm 16^\circ$(range 30–60°). The angle between the QRS and the delta wave frontal plane axis was $24^\circ \pm 15^\circ$. The R/S ratio in lead III was greater than 1 in 4 patients, equal to 1 in two, and less than 1 in one patient. The delta wave was positive in the inferior leads and in V_5 and V_6 in all patients (Fig. 6.1). The QRS transition (R/S $>$ 1) in the precordial leads occurred in lead V_2 in 5 patients, in V_3 in one, and in V_4 in one. Patients 6 and 7 had an ECG pattern indistinguishable from a midseptal bypass tract located at the apical region of the triangle of Koch (Fig. 6.2). Patient 1 had a positive delta wave in lead V_1, suggestive of a left-sided ventricular insertion, whereas all the others had a flat or negative delta wave in lead V_1, consistent with a right ventricular insertion.

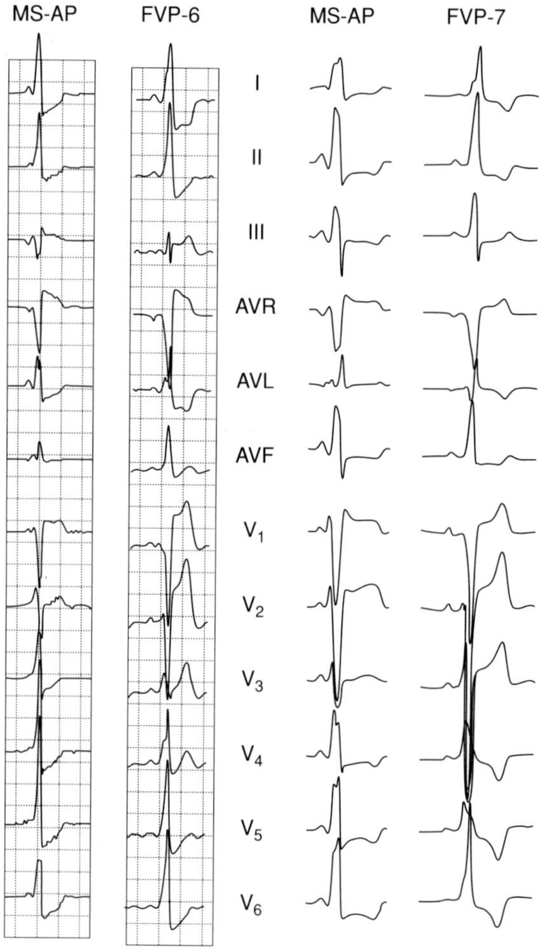

Figure 6.2 ECGs of patients 6 and 7 with an FV pathways (FVP) showing a broad QRS complex. They are displayed for comparison with the ECGs of 2 group III patients with midseptal bypass tracts (MS-AP).

Electrophysiological evaluation

The mean AH and HV intervals were 62 ± 10 ms and 24 ± 3 ms, respectively. During right or left atrial extrastimulation, all patients responded with prolongation of the AH interval with a fixed HV interval. In 3 of 7 patients (42%), a critically timed atrial premature beat blocked in the FV pathway, causing prolongation of the HV interval and normalization of the QRS complex (Fig. 6.3). The electrocardiogram during AVNRT showed a wide QRS tachycardia due to bystander anterograde conduction over a FV pathway in case 7 (Fig. 6.4).

All patients received intravenous adenosine as a bolus and responded with prolongation of the PR interval (AH interval) without changing the degree of

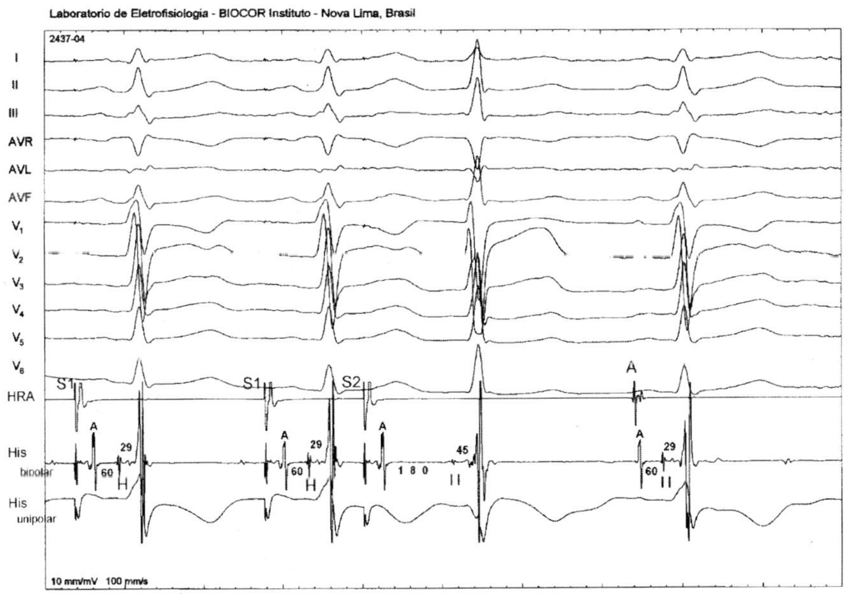

Figure 6.3 Case 5. A critically timed atrial premature beat blocked in the FV pathway and conducted with a normal HV interval and without ventricular preexcitation. Shown are recordings from surface leads and intracardiac electrograms from the high lateral right atrium (HRA), a bipolar recording of the His bundle potential (His bipolar), and a unipolar recording from the distal electrode (His unipolar). Recording speed is 100 mm/s.

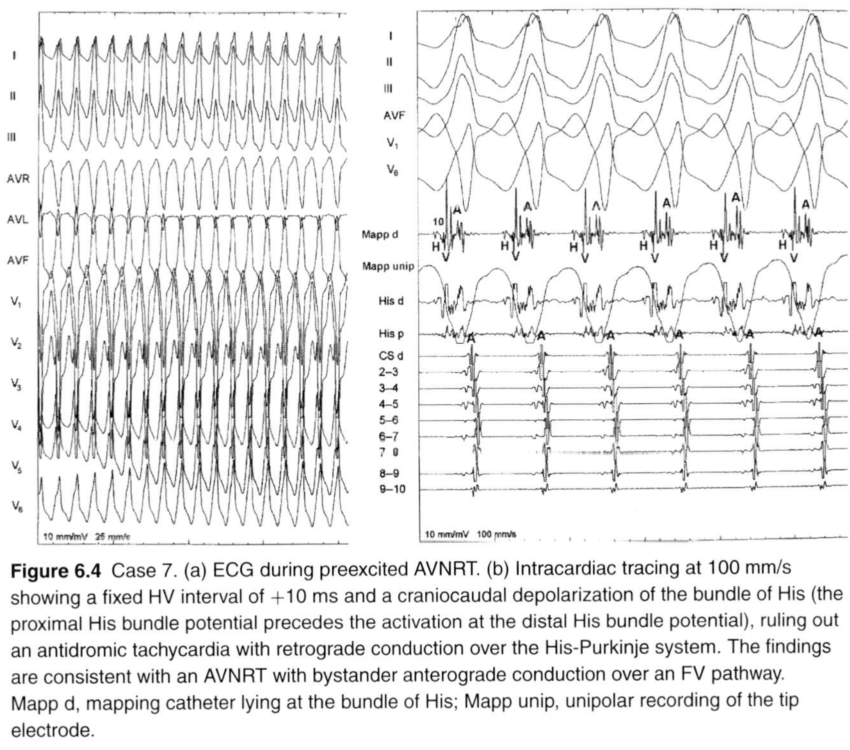

Figure 6.4 Case 7. (a) ECG during preexcited AVNRT. (b) Intracardiac tracing at 100 mm/s showing a fixed HV interval of +10 ms and a craniocaudal depolarization of the bundle of His (the proximal His bundle potential precedes the activation at the distal His bundle potential), ruling out an antidromic tachycardia with retrograde conduction over the His-Purkinje system. The findings are consistent with an AVNRT with bystander anterograde conduction over an FV pathway. Mapp d, mapping catheter lying at the bundle of His; Mapp unip, unipolar recording of the tip electrode.

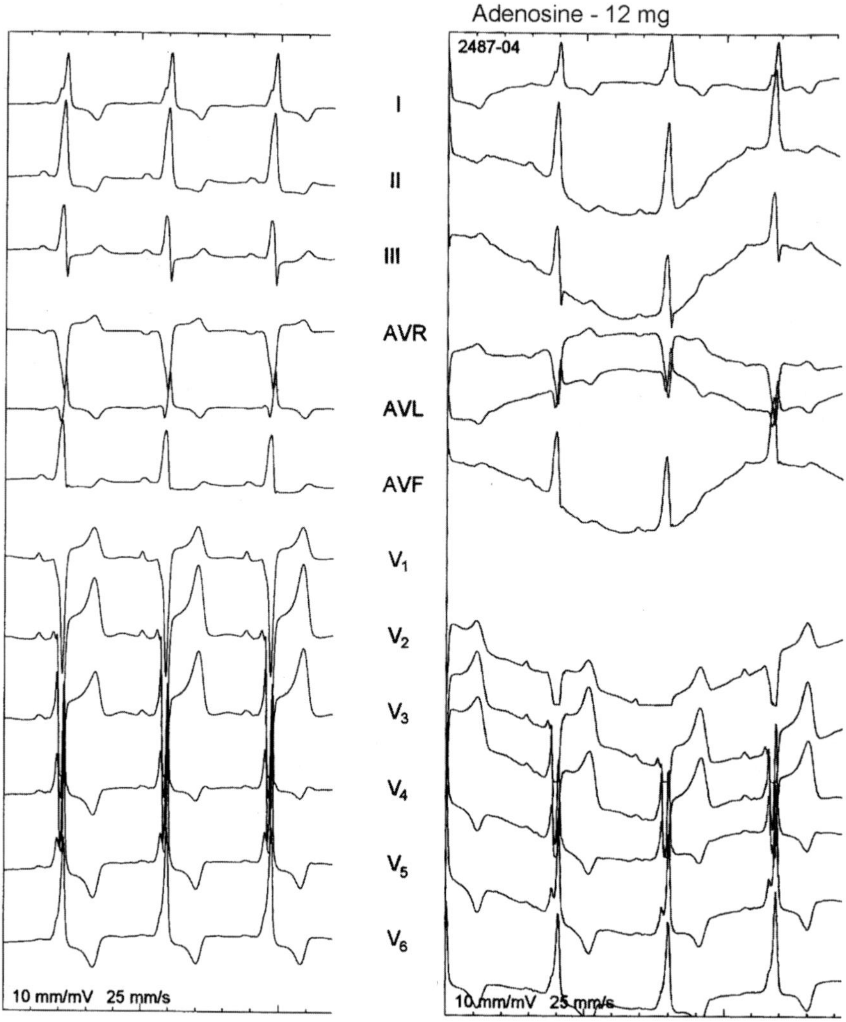

Figure 6.5 Case 7. The 12-lead ECG before and after an IV bolus of adenosine, showing prolongation of the PR interval without affecting the amount of ventricular preexcitation.

preexcitation (and the HV interval). Atrial beats conducted under adenosine infusion always showed preexcitation (Fig. 6.5).

Groups of patients with accessory AV pathways (Table 6.2)

1 *QRS axis in the frontal plane.* Midseptal AP -15° to $+60^\circ$ (mean $32^\circ \pm 22^\circ$); anteroseptal AP 0° to $+75^\circ$ (mean $45^\circ \pm 25^\circ$).

2 *Delta wave axis in the frontal plane.* Midseptal and anteroseptal AP had an intermediate delta wave axis: 0–60° (mean $23^\circ \pm 18^\circ$) and 0–60° (mean $43^\circ \pm 18^\circ$), respectively.

3 *Angle between the QRS and the delta wave axis*. Midseptal 10–40° (mean 23° ± 8°); anteroseptal accessory pathway 0–15° (mean 4° ± 8°) ($p < 0.0001$, compared with group I patients).
4 *QRS width*. The mean QRS width in the 40 patients with accessory AV pathways was 0.14 ± 0.01 ($p < 0.0001$, compared with the group I patients).
5 *R/S ratio in lead III*. Seven of the 20 patients with midseptal AP had an R/S ratio equal to 1 in lead III; the same ratio was less than 1 in the remaining 13 patients. All 7 patients with midseptal accessory pathways with an R/S ration of 1 had their AP located in the apical part of the triangle of Koch, just below the bundle of His. In all patients with anteroseptal AP, the R/S ratio in lead III was greater than 1.
6 *Delta wave negativity in inferior leads*. Midseptal accessory pathways showed positive delta waves in lead III in 12 of the 20 patients and a negative delta wave in lead III in 8 of 20. All 20 patients with anteroseptal AP showed positive delta waves in the inferior leads.
7 *Precordial lead transition to an R/S ratio greater than 1*. Midseptal AP: 5 patients showed R/S ratio greater than 1 in V_2, 11 in V_3, and 4 in V_4. Anteroseptal AP showed a shift to an R/S ratio of greater than 1, mainly in V_4 (16 of 20 patients) and less often in V_3 (4 patients).

Discussion

The septal region is a complex anatomic region harboring not only the FV pathways but approximately 30% of all accessory AV pathways. As a result, it is expected that the ECG presentation of the FV pathway may share some characteristics with septal AV pathways. If we apply previously published algorithms in the differential diagnosis of septal accessory pathways in patients with FV pathways, then these will be categorized as anteroseptal or midseptal bypass tracts [15, 16].

Patients with FV pathways show a variable PR interval. Some authors [3] describe a normal or short PR interval. Gallagher *et al.* [7] reported six patients with FV pathways with a PR interval of less than 0.12 s and electrophysiological evidence of enhanced AV nodal conduction. In our series the mean PR interval was 0.10 ± 0.01 (range 0.09–0.12) s, but no patient had enhanced AV nodal conduction.

Previous studies [12, 13] concentrated on the QRS configuration and delta wave morphology in lead V_1, which in our cohort showed a wide variability. According to our findings, FV pathways have overlapping ECG features with both anteroseptal and midseptal accessory bypass tracts. The mean QRS and delta wave frontal plane axis was normal in all three groups.

Electrocardiographic similarities with anteroseptal accessory pathways

The R/S ratio in lead III was greater than 1 in 4 of the 7 patients (57%) with FV pathways and in 100% of the patients with an anteroseptal AP ($p =$ ns). In contrast, patients with midseptal accessory pathways never showed an R/S ratio greater than 1.

Patients with FV pathways and patients with anteroseptal bypass tracts never showed a negative delta wave in inferior leads, in contrast with 25% of the patients with a midseptal accessory pathway.

ECG similarities with midseptal accessory pathways

Patients with FV pathways and patients with a midseptal bypass tract had a similar angle between the QRS and the delta wave axis in the frontal plane ($24^\circ \pm 15^\circ$ and $23^\circ \pm 8^\circ$, respectively) compared with the angle of $4^\circ \pm 8^\circ$ in patients with an anteroseptal bypass tract ($p < 0.0001$).

ECG dissimilarities between FV, midseptal, and anteroseptal accessory pathways

The transition to an R/S ratio of greater than 1 in the precordial leads occurred mainly in V_2 in patients with FV pathways, in V_3 in those with midseptal pathways, and in V_4 in those with anteroseptal bypass tracts.

The major feature differentiating FV pathways from a septal bypass tract was the QRS width: 0.12 ± 0.02 ms in the former and 0.14 ± 0.008 and 0.14 ± 0.01 ms in midseptal and anteroseptal bypass tracts, respectively ($p < 0.0001$).

The electrocardiogram during sinus rhythm in patients with FV pathways will show a short PR interval, usually with a minimal preexcitation pattern with a QRS width of 0.12 s, a normal frontal plane QRS and delta wave axis, a short angle between the QRS and the delta wave axis, and a precordial transition to an R/S ratio of greater than 1 most likely in V_2. It is worth mentioning that no patient with an anteroseptal or a midseptal bypass tract had minimal preexcitation.

Patients with left-sided bypass tracts may show minimal preexcitation. According to Bogun *et al.* [17] an rsR′ is usually found in lead V_6 in these patients, in contrast with an R pattern found in our eight patients with FV pathways. Fibers of the atriofascicular variety usually show minimal preexcitation, but an rS pattern can be found in lead III [18], while FV pathways usually show an R/S ratio of greater than 1 in lead III.

Clinical implications

FV pathways are responsible for a variable preexcitation pattern on surface electrocardiogram, as shown in this study. The ECG is similar to that of patients with anteroseptal and midseptal accessory AV pathways. A negative test with intravenous adenosine calls for an electrophysiological study for a correct diagnosis. It has been shown that FV pathways may be associated with other arrhythmogenic substrates, such as dual AV nodal pathways or rapidly conducting AV bypass tracts, and involved as bystanders during supraventricular tachycardia, causing ECG patterns of difficult interpretation, as shown in Fig. 6.4.

Conclusion

The ECGs of patients with FV pathways are similar to the ECGs of those with anteroseptal accessory pathways and midseptal bypass tracts located at the apex of the triangle of Koch, but the QRS is usually narrower and shows minimal preexcitation. FV pathways with a large QRS complex cannot be reliably differentiated from an anteroseptal or a midseptal bypass tract by the 12-lead surface ECG.

The definite diagnosis requires an intracardiac study observing the presence or absence of changes in the QRS complex during single test atrial stimulation and atrial pacing at increasing rates. This should always be done when ablation of septally located accessory pathways is considered.

Limitations

The main limitation to our study relates to the fact that the FV pathways were not ablated, and on the basis of the finding of an earliest ventricular activation close the bundle of His, we assume that they have a ventricular septum connection. The number of patients with FV pathways is so small that we cannot come to a definite conclusion.

Illustrative cases

We will present four selected cases to highlight the difficulties encountered by the cardiologist dealing with patients with palpitations, a likely preexcitation syndrome, and a complex ECG pattern. In this situation, often more than one accessory pathway is present.

Case 1

A 13-year-old male patient with the Wolff–Parkinson–White (WPW) syndrome and recurrent paroxysmal tachycardia was referred for catheter ablation. The 12-lead ECG in rest (Fig. 6.6a) was suggestive of a combination of two anterograde preexcitation patterns (a left-sided lateral accessory pathway and a right-sided or anteroseptal accessory pathway). A preexcited tachycardia was induced during electrophysiological study (Fig. 6.6b). A right-sided bypass tract was thought to be responsible for anterograde conduction of the electrical impulse during tachycardia. A left free-wall bypass tract was used for ventriculoatrial (VA) conduction, as shown by an eccentric left-sided VA conduction pattern. Since it was not possible to advance ventricular activation by means of atrial premature beats during tachycardia, we became suspicious of bystander anterograde conduction over an accessory pathway. We decided to ablate the left lateral bypass tract. Figure 6.6c shows the pattern of preexcitation after radiofrequency current ablation of the left free-wall pathway. After ablation there was no VA conduction. The AH interval was 60 milliseconds, the HV interval 25 milliseconds. Incremental atrial pacing increased the AH interval with the development of AV nodal Wenckebach at a cycle length of

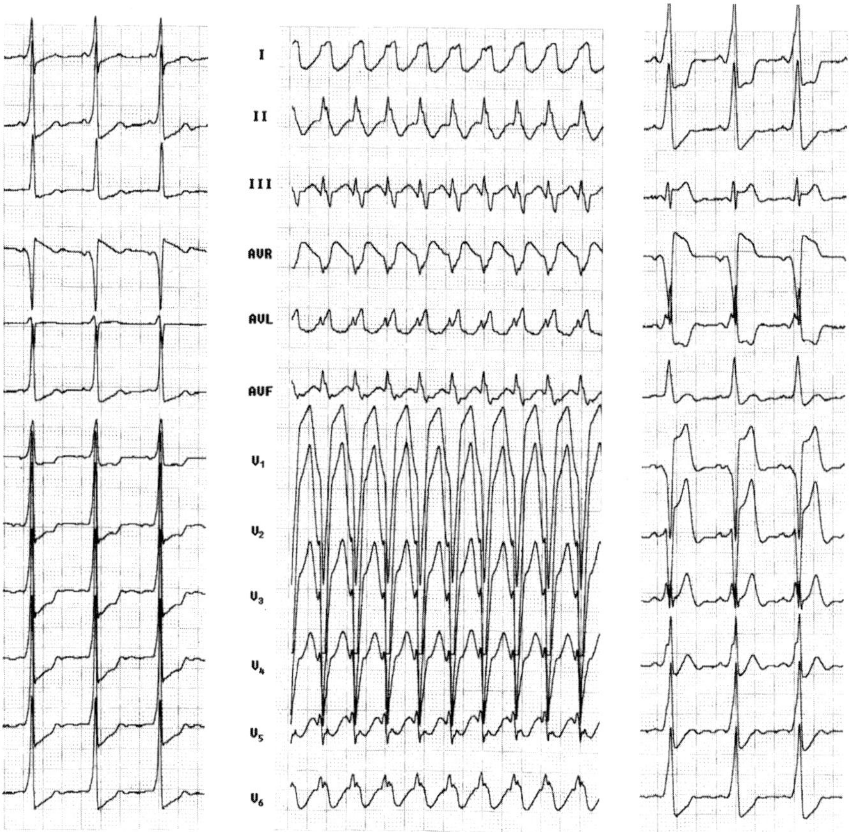

(a) (b) (c)

Figure 6.6 Case 1. (a) Baseline 12-lead ECG. The preexcitation pattern cannot be explained by a single accessory AV pathway (see text). (b) The QRS complex during the induced preexcited tachycardia resembles the QRS complex after ablation of the left-sided AP. (c) ECG after ablation of the left-sided accessory pathway (AP), showing a ventricular preexcitation pattern suggestive of a right-sided insertion of the accessory connection.

320 milliseconds. The effective refractory period of the AV node was 260 ms. The amount of right-sided preexcitation as well as the HV interval remained unchanged during atrial premature beats (Fig. 6.7). Intravenous adenosine infusion caused complete transient AV block without escape beats. No preexcited QRS complex occurred till AV conduction resumed. These findings are in agreement with an FV pathway inserting into the right ventricle, and no further ablation was attempted. The patient remained asymptomatic during a follow-up of three years.

Case 2

This 19-year-old male patient complained of palpitations but denied the occurrence of a sustained tachycardia. The 12-lead ECG showed preexcitation with

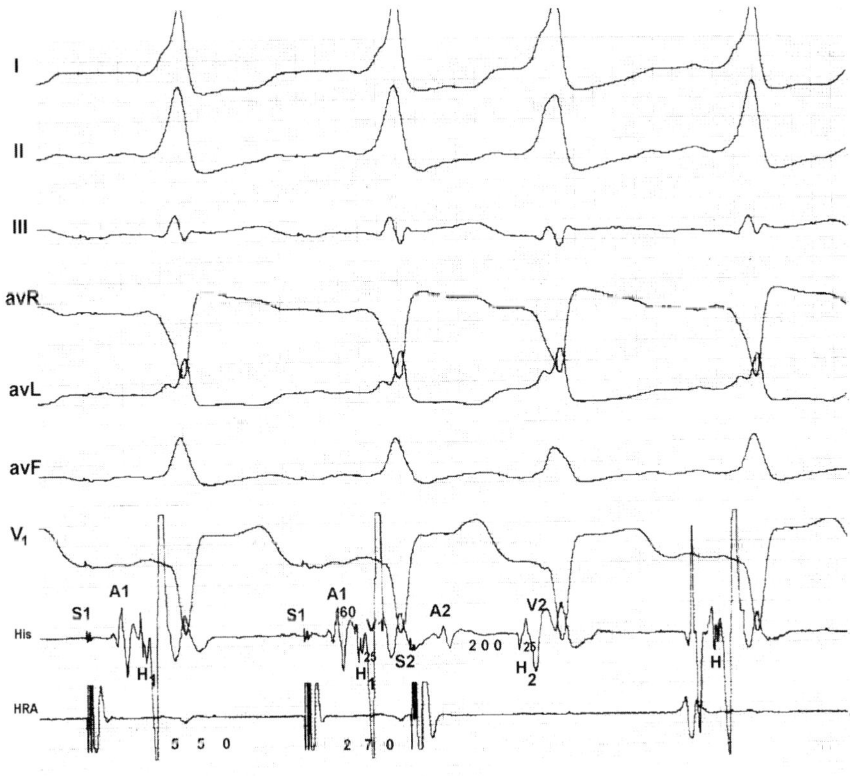

Figure 6.7 Case 1. An atrial premature beat with an interval of 270 ms is conducted with a long AH interval (200 ms) without changing the degree of ventricular preexcitation and the HV interval.

a P-delta interval of 0.12 s. His general practitioner referred him for electrophysiological evaluation. The delta wave was negative in V_1 and +60° in the frontal plane, consistent with an anteroseptal location of the accessory pathway (Fig. 6.8). The baseline AH interval was 50 ms, suggesting enhanced AV nodal conduction, but the AH conduction curve during incremental atrial pacing showed AH prolongation with an AV nodal Wenckebach conduction pattern at an atrial pacing cycle length of 380 ms. The HV interval was short (20 ms), did not change during atrial pacing, and showed a normal His bundle–right bundle activation sequence (Fig. 6.9). The amount of preexcitation did not change during atrial pacing at increasing rates and induced atrial fibrillation (Fig. 6.8). Ventricular pacing during sinus rhythm showed VA conduction, which was concentric and decremental. Intravenous adenosine was administered in sinus rhythm and during ventricular pacing. In both instances we observed complete conduction block. A few preexcited escape beats were recorded with the same QRS configuration as during sinus rhythm. No tachycardia could be induced by programmed stimulation. Mapping of ventricular activation during sinus

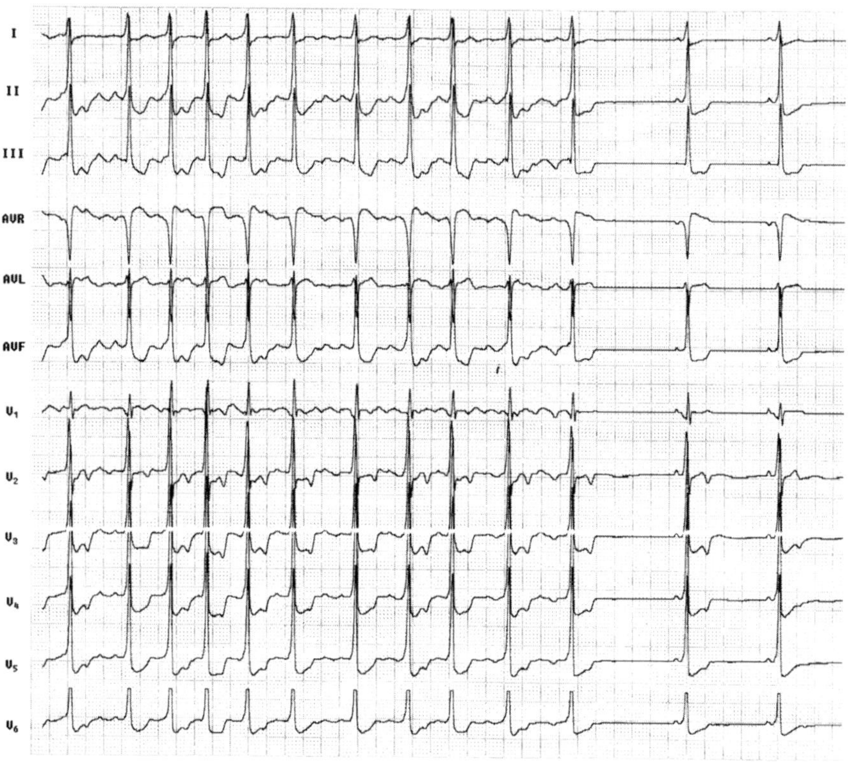

Figure 6.8 Case 2. An episode of self-terminating atrial fibrillation showing a "fixed degree" of preexcitation during atrial fibrillation and sinus rhythm. Note a delta wave configuration suggestive of an anteroseptal insertion of the accessory connection.

rhythm showed the shortest delta-V interval at the site of His bundle recording (Fig. 6.9). No ablation was attempted, and the patient was arrhythmia free during a six-month follow-up.

Case 3

A 19-year-old male patient with the WPW syndrome was admitted because of aborted sudden death while swimming. His sister underwent catheter ablation at the Biocor institute 2 years before because of multiple accessory pathways. The patient had frequent episodes of paroxysmal tachycardia before his collapse. The baseline 12-lead ECG (Fig. 6.10a) showed a ventricular preexcitation pattern that could not be explained by AV conduction over a single accessory pathway, suggesting the presence of multiple accessory pathways. During electrophysiological study a very fast antidromic AV tachycardia was induced by atrial extrastimuli (Fig. 6.10b). VA conduction during tachycardia showed long conduction time and midline atrial activation. During ventricular pacing,

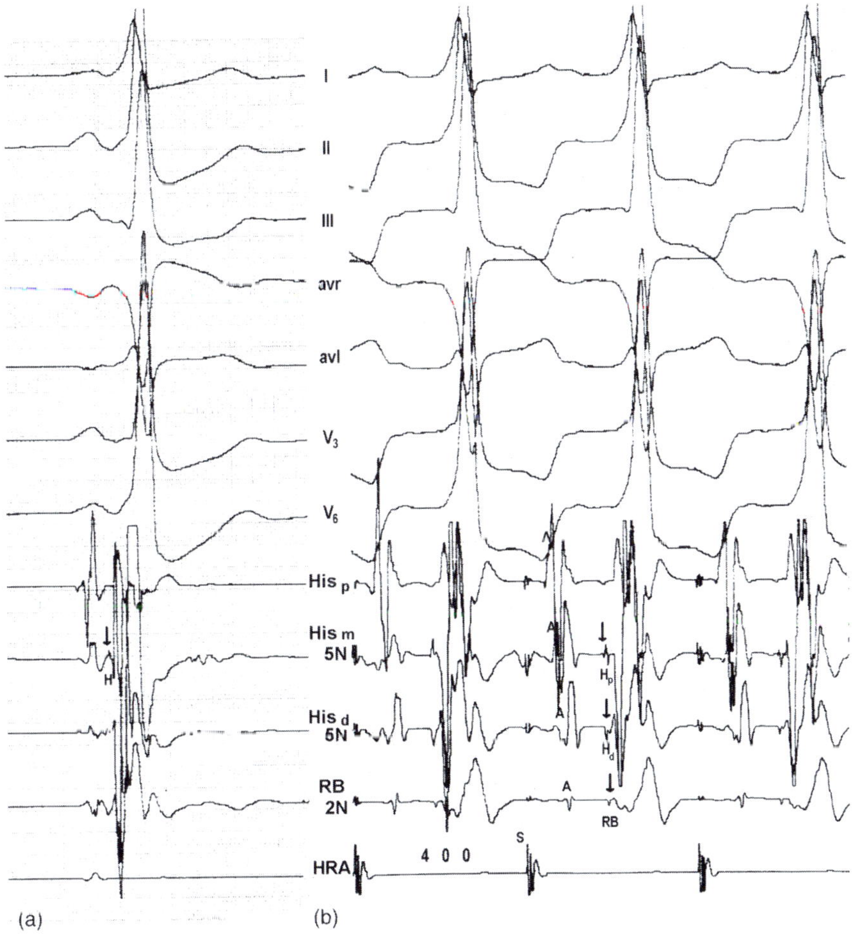

Figure 6.9 Case 2. (a) Sinus rhythm with preexcitation. (b) High right atrial stimulation (400 ms) showing prolongation of the AH interval with a fixed HV interval and similar degree of preexcitation as during sinus rhythm.

however, VA conduction was left sided. We decided to ablate this pathway, and we did it successfully by the transaortic approach. Following successful ablation of the left-sided accessory pathway, another pattern of ventricular preexcitation appeared (Fig. 6.10c). A midseptal accessory AV bypass tract with bidirectional conduction was also successfully ablated at the base of the triangle of Koch. After ablation of these two APs, preexcitation persisted but with a narrower QRS and a negative delta wave in V_1 (Fig. 6.10). Tachycardia could no longer be induced. The AH interval was short, but AV nodal conduction assessment showed a normal behavior during incremental atrial pacing and atrial premature stimuli. The HV interval was short and remained fixed during

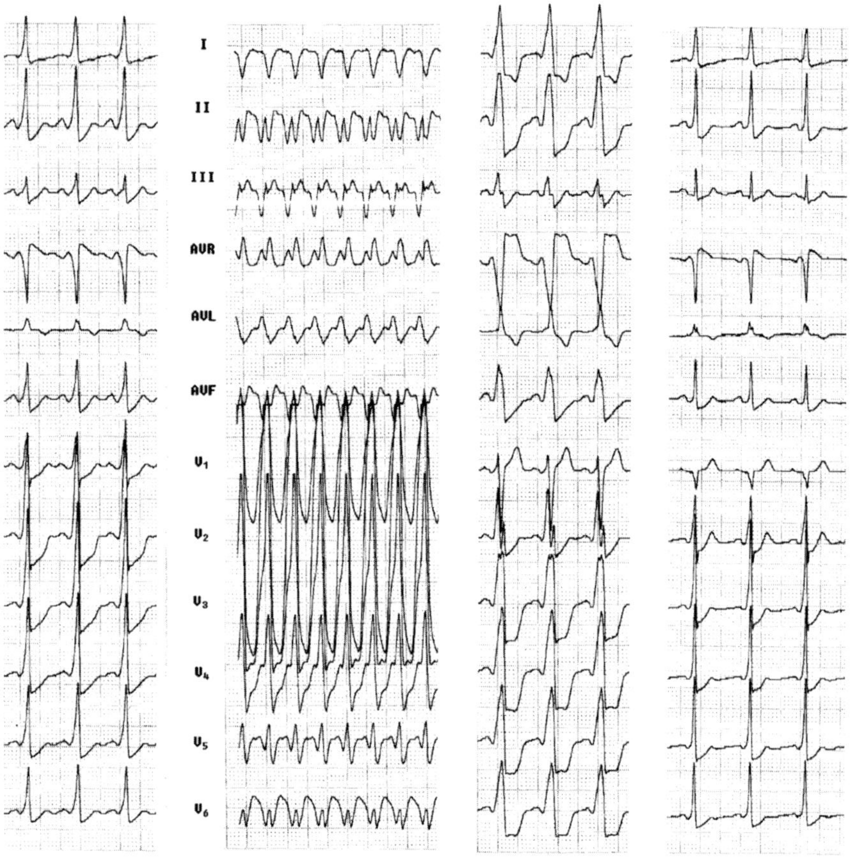

(a) (b) (c) (d)

Figure 6.10 Case 3. (a) The 12-lead ECG with a delta axis in the frontal plane at 60° with a discordant delta axis in the horizontal plane suggesting multiple accessory AV pathways. (b) Antidromic tachycardia anterogradely using two accessory pathways (a right midseptal and a left free-wall AP) for anterograde conduction. (c) After ablating the left-sided AP, the 12-lead ECG is compatible with a right midseptal AP. (d) After ablating the midseptal AP, the ECG still shows ventricular preexcitation in the anteroseptal area, but with less preexcitation.

incremental atrial pacing, and so did the amount of ventricular preexcitation. Response to intravenous adenosine was 2:1 AV block during sinus rhythm (Fig. 6.11) without any change in the QRS configuration. The diagnosis of an FV pathway inserting in the right anteroseptal area was made. The patient was free of arrhythmias during a one-year follow-up.

Case 4

A 51-year-old asymptomatic male patient was referred for electrophysiological evaluation, because he showed ventricular preexcitation during a routine preoperative examination. The rest 12-lead ECG (Fig. 6.11a) showed a short PR interval (0–10 s) and minimal preexcitation with an RBBB-like pattern suggestive of a left-sided accessory pathway. Atrial activation pattern during right ventricular pacing was concentric, with decremental VA conduction. Incremental atrial pacing at the coronary sinus ostium resulted in prolongation of the AH interval but no change in the HV interval and the degree of preexcitation.

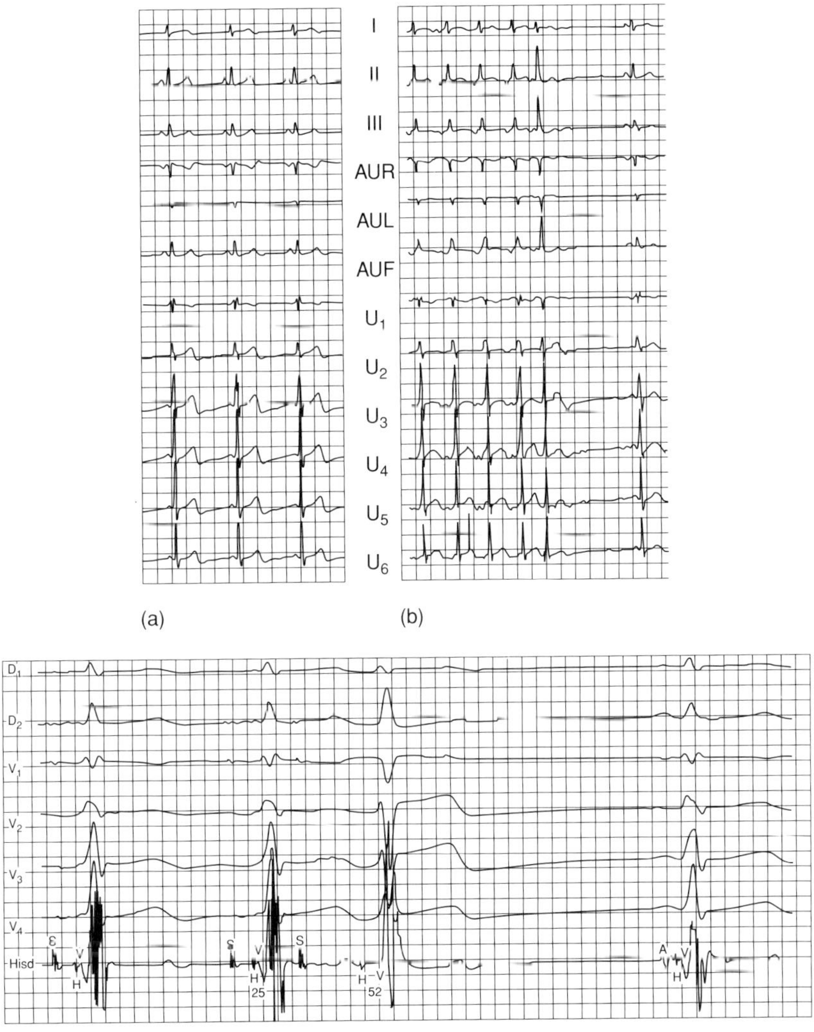

Figure 6.11 Case 4. (a) The 12-lead ECG showing sinus rhythm, a short PR interval, and a QRS configuration consistent with minimal left-sided preexcitation. (b) Coronary sinus pacing did not increase the degree of preexcitation. An atrial premature beat narrows the QRS complex by conduction block of the FV pathway. (c) A 240-ms coupled atrial premature beat delivered at the coronary sinus ostium narrows the QRS complex with normalization of the HV interval, suggesting block of the FV pathway.

Atrial premature beats with a coupling interval below 300 ms showed a normal HV interval followed by a narrow QRS complex (Fig. 6.11 right panel). These complexes were also seen at short RR intervals during induced atrial fibrillation. Intravenous adenosine (up to 36 μg) did not cause AV block; it resulted in sinus bradycardia and a junctional rhythm with a preexcited QRS complex. An FV pathway inserting in the left ventricle was the likely diagnosis, and catheter ablation was not performed.

Enhanced AV nodal conduction was a common finding among the patients studied by Gallagher *et al.* [7]. However, our 4 patients, in spite of having a short intranodal conduction time (AH interval) during sinus rhythm, showed normal AH interval lengthening and AV nodal behavior during incremental atrial pacing. For all our 4 patients, the classic electrophysiological findings of an FV connection during incremental atrial pacing include prolongation of the AH interval without changes in the HV interval, a constant degree of preexcitation, and a fixed relationship between the His bundle and the right bundle potential.

We found that intravenous adenosine was very useful as a method to assess the relationship between the FV pathway and its connection to the AV node–His bundle system. The use of adenosine triphosphate as a diagnostic tool is based on its transient, markedly negative AV nodal dromotropic effects [19]. In addition, adenosine shortens the action potential duration of an accessory pathway [20]. Adenosine did not produce a greater degree of preexcitation in any of our patients but created second degree or complete AV block with junctional beats having the same degree of preexcitation and a short HV interval as during sinus rhtyhm. His bundle pacing producing an identical QRS as during sinus rhythm is another method to demonstrate the presence of an FV fiber.

Two of our patients had associated bypass tracts and circus movement tachycardias. Gallagher *et al.* [7] reported an associated WPW syndrome in 1 out of their 6 patients, Sallee III *et al.* [10] found multiple accessory pathways in one out of their three children, and the patient reported by Kottkamp *et al.* [8] also had a left lateral bypass tract. The child reported by Ganz *et al.* [9] did not have associated WPW. Taking all these patients with FV pathways together, including ours [4, 5], the incidence of associated WPW comes to 39% (7 out of 18 patients). Multiple accessory pathways are estimated to occur in up to 13% of WPW patients [21]. Higher figures may represent bias due to referral of symptomatic patients. Nonetheless, in patients with ventricular preexcitation referred for catheter ablation, it is important to recognize that an FV pathway and not an anteroseptal bypass tract is present, avoiding damage to the AV node–His bundle system if such a pathway is mistakenly targeted for catheter ablation.

Summary

One should be especially suspicious for an additional FV pathway when the findings on the 12-lead ECG during sinus rhythm cannot be explained by ventricular preexcitation over one accessory AV pathway only. We ablated the left-sided pathways first (cases 1 and 3) and then the midseptal accessory pathway (case 3) after having obtained electrophysiological data supporting their location and their active role during tachycardia. After ablation of these pathways, the remaining preexcitation should be assessed carefully.

References

1 Mahaim I, Benatt A. Nouvelles recherches sur les connexions supérieures de la branch gauche du faisceau de His-Tawara avec cloison interventriculaire. *Cardiologia* 1938;1:61.

2 Wellens HJJ. *Electrical Stimulation of the Heart in the Study and Treatment of Tachycardias.* Baltimore: University Park Press; 1971:70.

3 Josephson ME. Preexcitation syndromes. In: Josephson ME, ed. *Clinical Cardiac Electrophysiology: Techniques and Interpretations.* Philadelphia: Lippincott Williams & Wilkins; 2002:419.

4 Sternick EB, Gerken LM, Vrandecic M, Wellens HJJ. Fasciculoventricular pathways. *J Cardiovasc Electrophysiol* 2003;14:1057.

5 Sternick EB, Rodriguez LM, Gerken LM, Wellens HJJ. The electrocardiogram of patients with fasciculoventricular pathways. A comparative study with patients with anteroseptal and midseptal accessory pathways. *Heart Rhythm* 2005;2:1.

6 Lev M, Fox SM, Bharati S, *et al*: Mahaim and James fibers as a basis for a unique variety of ventricular preexcitation. *Am J Cardiol* 1975;36:880.

7 Gallagher JJ, Smith WM, Kasell JH, *et al*. Role of Mahaim fibers in cardiac arrhythmias in man. *Circulation* 1981;64:176.

8 Kottkamp H, Hindricks G, Shenasa H, *et al*. Variants of preexcitation-specialized atriofascicular pathways, nodofascicular pathways, and fasciculoventricular pathways: electrophysiologic findings and target sites for radiofrequency catheter ablation. *J Cardiovasc Electrophysiol* 1996;7:916.

9 Ganz LI, Elson JJ, Chenarides JG. Preexcitation in a child with syncope. Where is the connection? *J Cardiovasc Electrophysiol* 1998;9:892.

10 Sallee III D, Van Hare GF. Preexcitation secondary to fasciculoventricular pathway in children: a report of three cases. *J Cardiovascular Electrophysiol* 1999;10:36.

11 Oh S, Choi YS, Choi EK, *et al*: Electrocardiographic characteristics of Fasciculoventricular pathways. *Pacin Clin Electrophysiol* 2004;28:25.

12 Myaguchi K, Tsuzuki J, Yokota M, Hayashi H. Characteristic findings on the standard 12-lead ECG in patients with the fasciculoventricular Mahaim fiber. *J Electrocardiol* 1992;25:253.

13 Ito M, Onodera S, Noshiro H, *et al*. Effect of class IA antiarrhythmic agents on fasciculoventricular fibers. *J Electrocardiol* 1990;23:323.

14 Rodriguez LM, Smeets JL, de Chillou C, *et al*. The 12-lead electrocardiogram in midseptal, anteroseptal, posteroseptal and right free wall accessory pathways. Am *J Cardiol* 1993;72:1274.

15 Fitzpatrick AP, Gonzales RP, Lesh MD, *et al*. New algorithm for the localization of accessory atrioventricular connections using a baseline electrocardiogram. *J Am Coll Cardiol* 1994;23:107.

16 Arruda MS, McClelland JH, Wang X, *et al*. Development and validation of an ECG algorithm for identifying accessory pathway ablation site in the Wolff–Parkinson–White syndrome. *J Cardiovasc Electrophysiol* 1998;9:2.

17 Bogun F, Kalusche D, Li YG, *et al*. Septal Q waves in surface electrocardiographic lead V6 exclude minimal ventricular preexcitation. Am *J Cardiol* 1999;84:101.
18 Sternick EB, Timmermans C, Sosa EA, *et al*. The electrocardiogram in sinus rhythm and tachycardia in patients with Mahaim fibers. The importance of an "rS" pattern in lead III. *J Am Coll Cardiol* 2004; 44:1626.
19 Belhassen B. Adenosine triphosphate in cardiac arrhytmias: from therapeutic to diagnostic use. *Pacin Clin Electrophysiol* 2000;25:98.
20 Garrat CJ, Griffith MJ, O'Nunain S, *et al*. Effects of intravenous adenosine on antegrade refractoriness of accessory atrioventricular connections. *Circulation* 1991;84:1962.
21 Colavita PG, Packer DL, Pressley JC, *et al*. Frequency, diagnosis and clinical characteristics of patients with multiple accessory atrioventricular pathways. Am *J Cardiol* 1987;59:601.

CHAPTER 7

Conduction disturbances in accessory pathways

Rapidly conducting accessory pathways

Accessory atrioventricular (AV) bypass tracts are myocardial bridges that connect the atrium with the ventricle. Variations among the tricuspid and the mitral annulus structure may account for some anatomic differences between right and left-sided bypass tracts. The mitral annulus consists of a complete fibrous ring, and left-sided accessory pathways are usually composed of thin strands of myocardium. In contrast, the tricuspid ring, which is larger, can have "gaps," by which myocardium from the atrium and the ventricle can connect. Right-sided bypass tracts consist of small or broad bands of muscle [1, 2]. These right- and left-sided myocardial bridges, either broad or small, have a characteristic all-or-none impulse conduction pattern. During rapid atrial pacing there is conduction without delay and sudden block. Conduction time to and through a bypass tract will depend on its location, its structure, and the quality of the input of the impulse. For example, when the site of impulse formation is far from the atrial end of the accessory pathway, a longer PR interval and a smaller degree of preexcitation will result, and this does not mean that there is decremental conduction in the bypass tract.

Intermittent conduction over a rapidly conducting bypass tract is not uncommonly observed. The likely causes are a long refractory period of the bypass tract, phase 3 and phase 4 block in the accessory pathway, concealed anterograde conduction produced by premature beats, or an orthodromic tachycardia. Unapparent conduction over the accessory pathway during sinus rhythm, because the pathway is located far from the sinus node, must be differentiated from intermittent conduction, because in the former situation unlike in the latter a short anterograde refractory period of the bypass may be present and such patients may be at risk of sudden death if atrial fibrillation supervenes. Minimal ventricular preexcitation is typically observed in left free-wall accessory pathways because the degree of preexcitation is dependent on the intra-atrial conduction time from the sinus node to the accessory pathway and the conduction time through the AV node—His bundle branch system. Two electrocardiographic (ECG) signs suggest the presence of minimal preexcitation: the absence of a septal Q wave in lead V_6 [3] or the presence of a pseudo partial RBBB (rSr′) in lead V_1 [4].

Conduction through an accessory pathway may disappear over the years. Chen *et al.* [5] reported loss of anterograde conduction in one-fifth of symptomatic patients with Wolff–Parkinson–White (WPW) syndrome. Others reported even higher figures in children (50%) [6].

Decrementally conducting accessory pathways

Decremental conduction (prolonged P-delta wave) is defined as a rate-dependent prolongation of the accessory pathway conduction time to more than 30 ms. This has been documented in atriofascicular, nodofascicular, and nodoventricular pathways, and also in AV bypass tracts, which are usually located in the right anterior free wall but are occasionally found at the posterior mitral annulus (see Chapter 3). Other instances associated with decremental conduction are damaged rapidly conducting accessory pathways developing slow conduction after a previous unsuccessful catheter ablation [7], rapidly conducting bypass tracts with a tortuous course [8], and bypass tracts with specific distal insertion having a small to a larger cable configuration [9] (Fig. 7.1).

Slow conduction versus conduction disturbances

ECG recognition of the presence of an atriofascicular pathway can be hampered by the characteristic slow conduction, which results in a normal or a minimally

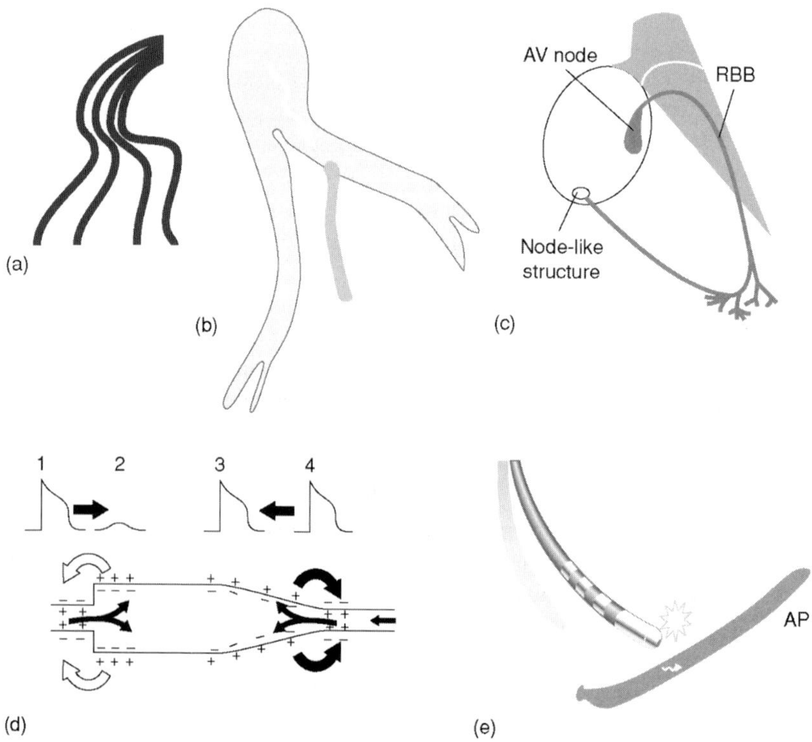

Figure 7.1 Substrates associated with decremental conduction: A, AP with a tortuous course; B, AP with a proximal end distal to the AV node; C, atriofascicular pathways; D, smaller to larger cable configuration (4-3); E, slow conduction in AP with a scar caused by a previous catheter ablation.

preexcited QRS complex due to a fusion with the conducted sinus impulse over the normal AV node–His–Purkinje axis. Extreme examples of slow conduction are the "latent" Mahaim fibers [10, 11], which are unable to conduct sinus impulses or paced atrial beats to the ventricle before ventricular activation over the AV node–His–Purkinje axis.

Another striking feature of decrementally conducting fibers is their incapability of impulse conduction in the retrograde ventriculoatrial (VA) direction. This is a common feature of all anterograde decrementally conducting accessory pathways, for which we have no explanation. Accepting that atriofascicular pathways have AV node-like tissue, by analogy with the conduction properties of the AV node, one should expect that retrograde conduction through a decrementally conducting accessory pathway would occur at a similar figure, 2/3 of the patients. There are very few case reports of anterogradely decrementally conducting fibers with VA conduction [12, 13]. In most cases the VA conduction can be explained by an additional concealed accessory pathway. Decremental conduction in one direction without conduction in the other direction is also found in "concealed" decrementally conduction accessory AV pathways. They conduct only from ventricle to atrium and not from atrium to ventricle [14].

Conduction disturbances in decrementally conducting fibers

First-degree intra-Mahaim "block" (latent Mahaim fiber conduction)

Some patients with Mahaim fibers have no anterograde conduction during sinus rhythm or atrial pacing but can still support an antidromic circus movement tachycardia. In some patients the conduction delay occurred in the distal part of the atriofascicular connection (long MV interval), while a proximal delay (long AM interval) was observed in others (Fig. 7.2). The likely explanation for the "latent" conduction might be that owing to the conduction delay in the decremental fiber, the ventricle could not be preexcited during sinus rhythm, because the AV node–His–Purkinje axis always has a faster conduction time. The main challenge in this situation is to correctly differentiate the antidromic tachycardia from a ventricular tachycardia with an LBBB-like configuration. It is noteworthy that antidromic tachycardia can only be induced with ventricular pacing in patients with a "latent" Mahaim. During tachycardia, a critically timed late atrial premature beat can advance or delay ventricular activation and be helpful in achieving the correct diagnosis of a decremental fiber. Such patients do not show ventricular preexcitation; however, during careful mapping at the annulus accessory pathway potentials (M potentials) can be found targeted for ablation [10, 11].

Second-degree intra-Mahaim block (spontaneous intermittent conduction and prolonged refractoriness)

We studied eight patients with the short AV Mahaim fibers (accessory AV pathways with decremental properties) and observed spontaneous conduction disturbances in two (25%) [15]. One of these patients showed intermittent

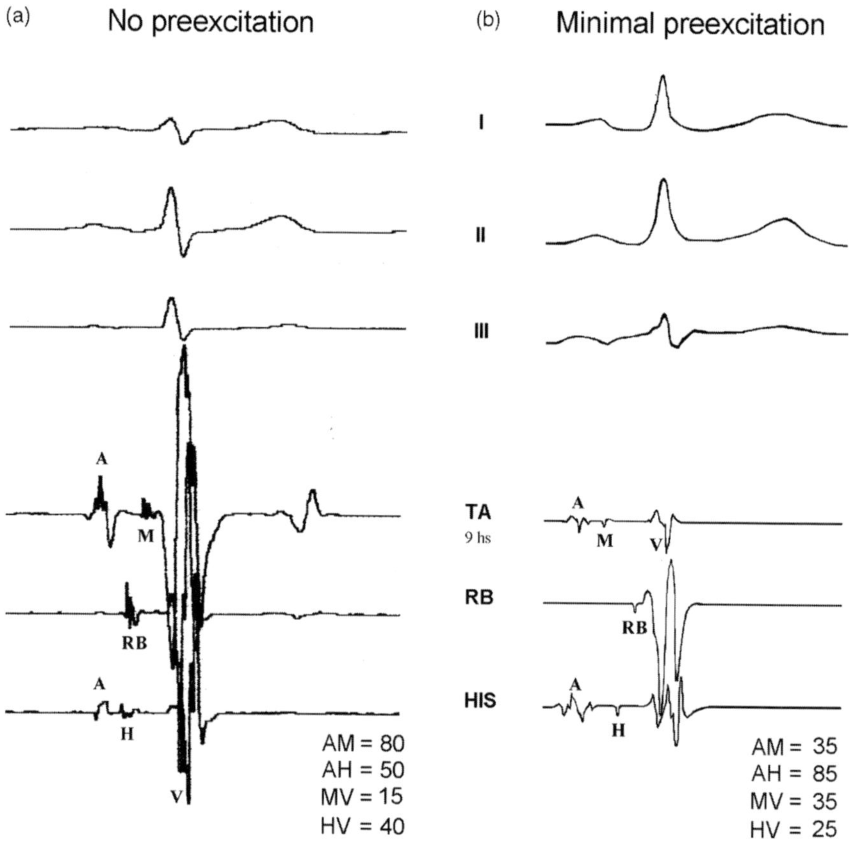

Figure 7.2 (a) A patient without preexcitation showing a longer AM + MV conduction time (95 ms) and a shorter AH + HV interval (90 ms). (b) A patient showing a shorter conduction time over the atriofascicular fiber than over the His–Purkinje system (70 vs. 110 ms), resulting in minimal preexcitation (rS pattern in lead III).

conduction over the decremental pathway (Figs 7.3 & 7.6), while the other had one-to-one AV conduction over the Mahaim fiber with a spontaneous second-degree Wenckebach-like block during isoproterenol infusion (Figs 7.4 & 7.5). The fiber in the patient with intermittent preexcitation had AV node-like properties, showing conduction block during adenosine infusion and Mahaim automaticity during radiofrequency current ablation. The other patient, however, did not respond to adenosine or showed automaticity during ablation. We have recently reported a patient with a nodoventricular fiber showing a very long refractory period. Its presence could not be recognized during sinus rhythm or during AV nodal reentrant tachycardia, which was the patient's clinical problem. However, during 2:1 AV nodal reentrant tachycardia, there was anterograde bystander conduction over the atriofascicular fiber (Figs 7.6 & 7.7) [16].

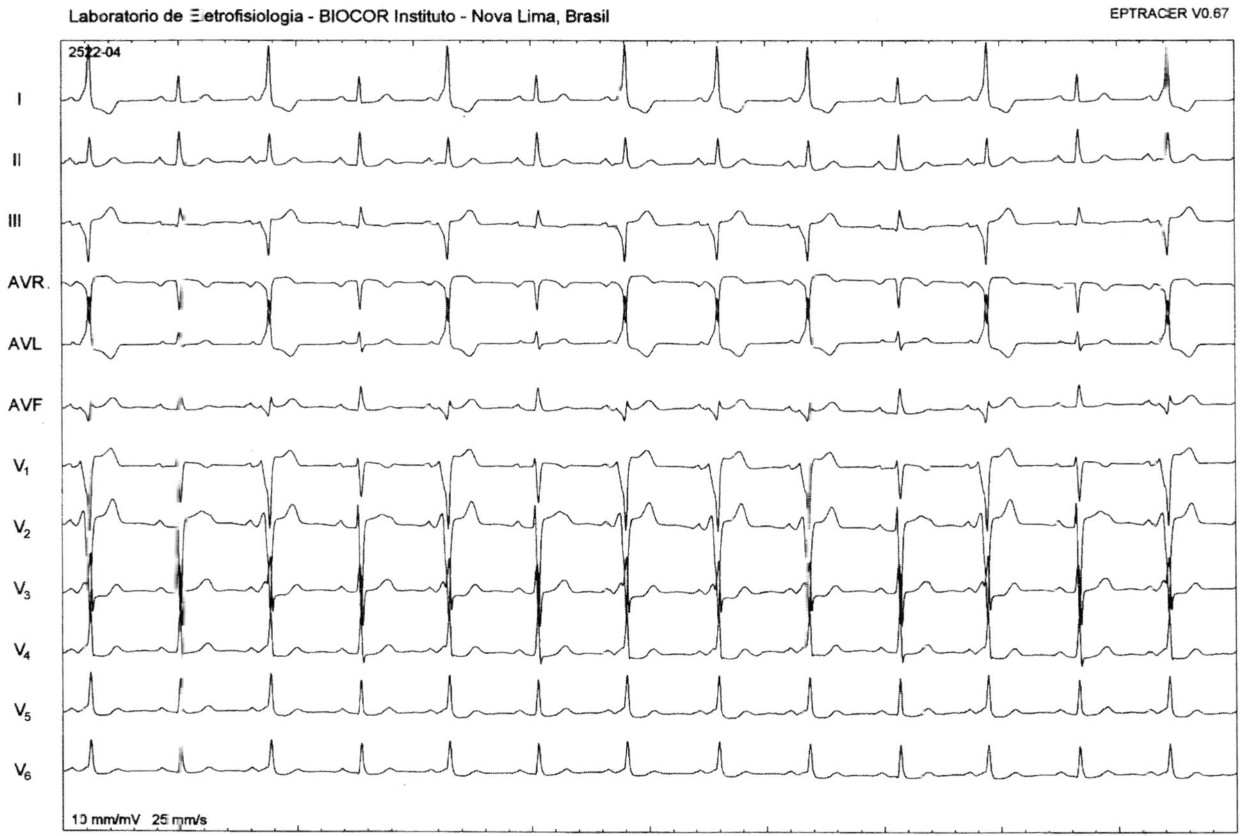

Figure 7.3 A 12-lead ECG during sinus rhythm with intermittent ventricular preexcitation over a right-sided decrementally conducting short AV pathway.

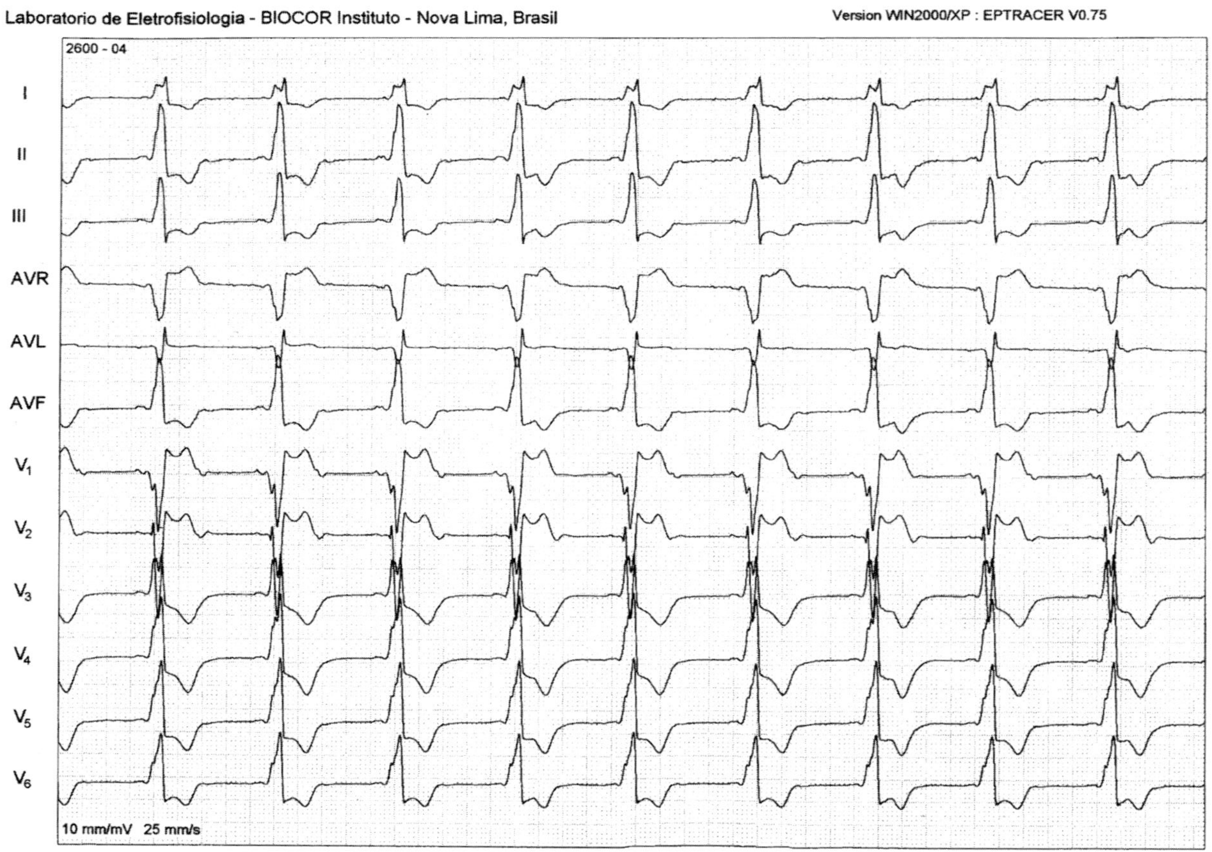

Figure 7.4 A 12-lead ECG showing sinus bradycardia with overt ventricular preexcitation over a decrementally conducting right anterior short AV pathway.

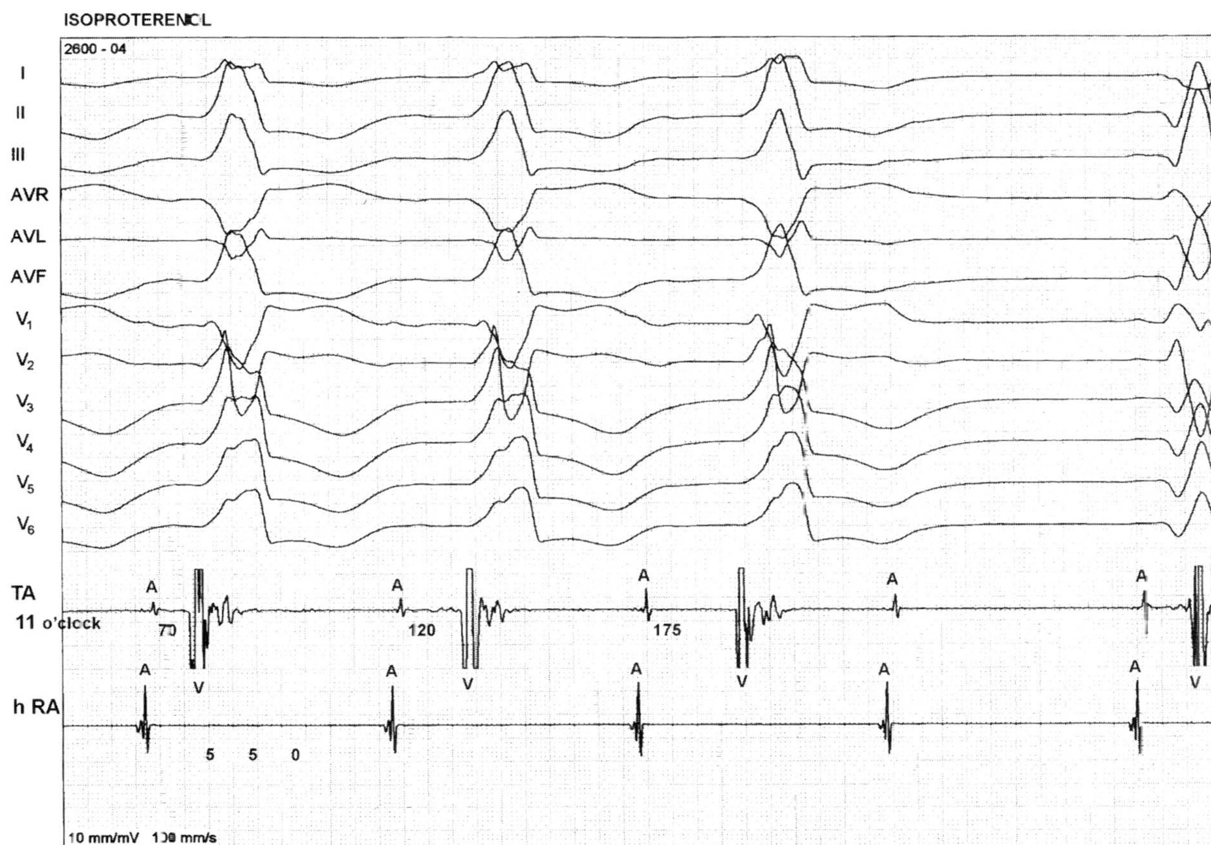

Figure 7.5 Same patient as Fig. 7.4 Wenckebach block in a short AV fiber during sinus rhythm under isoproterenol infusion. The ablation catheter (TA) recorded an early ventricular electrogram at the annulus. The recording speed was 100 mm/s.

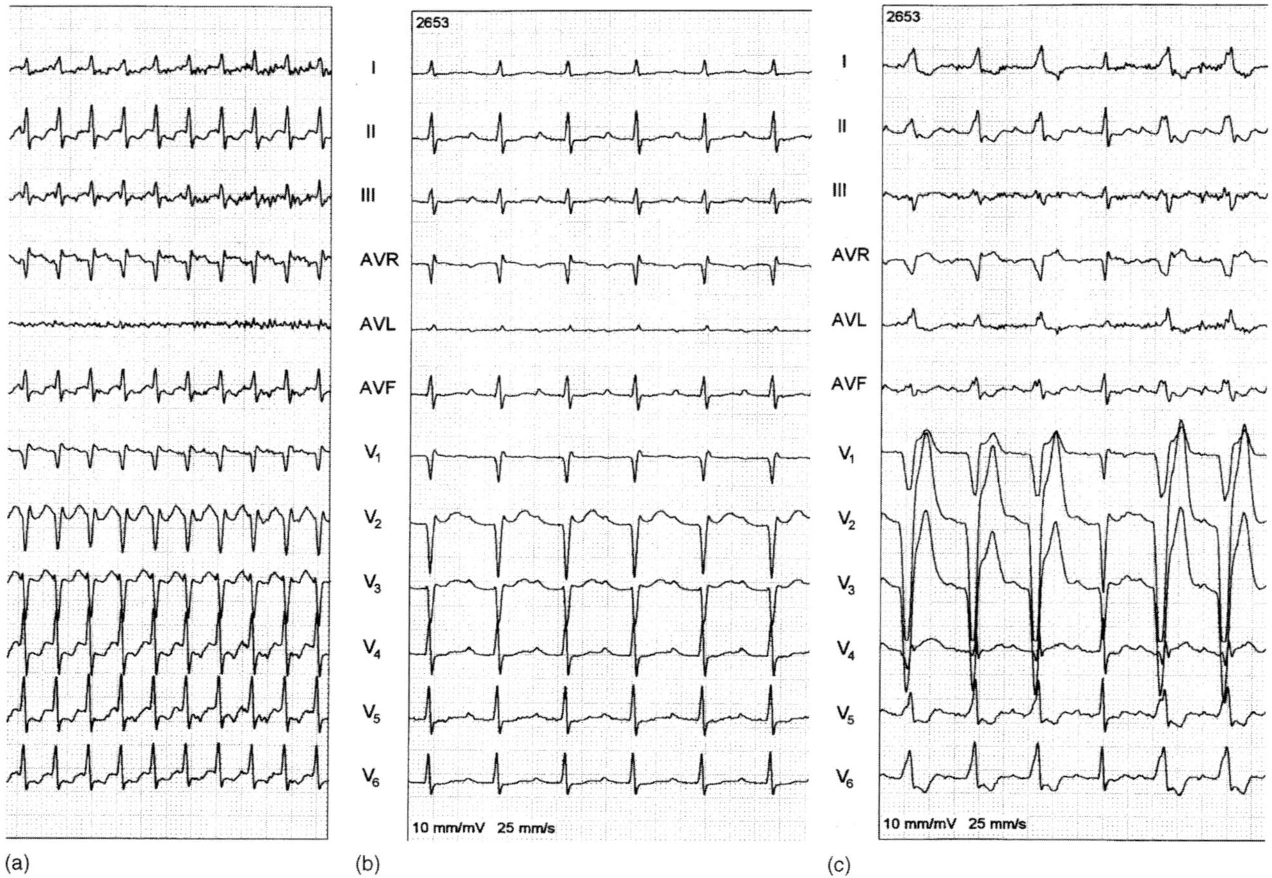

Figure 7.6 A 12-lead ECG: (a) narrow QRS tachycardia due to AV nodal reentry; (b) AVNRT with 2:1 block; (c) AVNRT with 2:1 block and bystander preexcitation over an atriofascicular fiber. The fourth QRS complex is not preexcited.

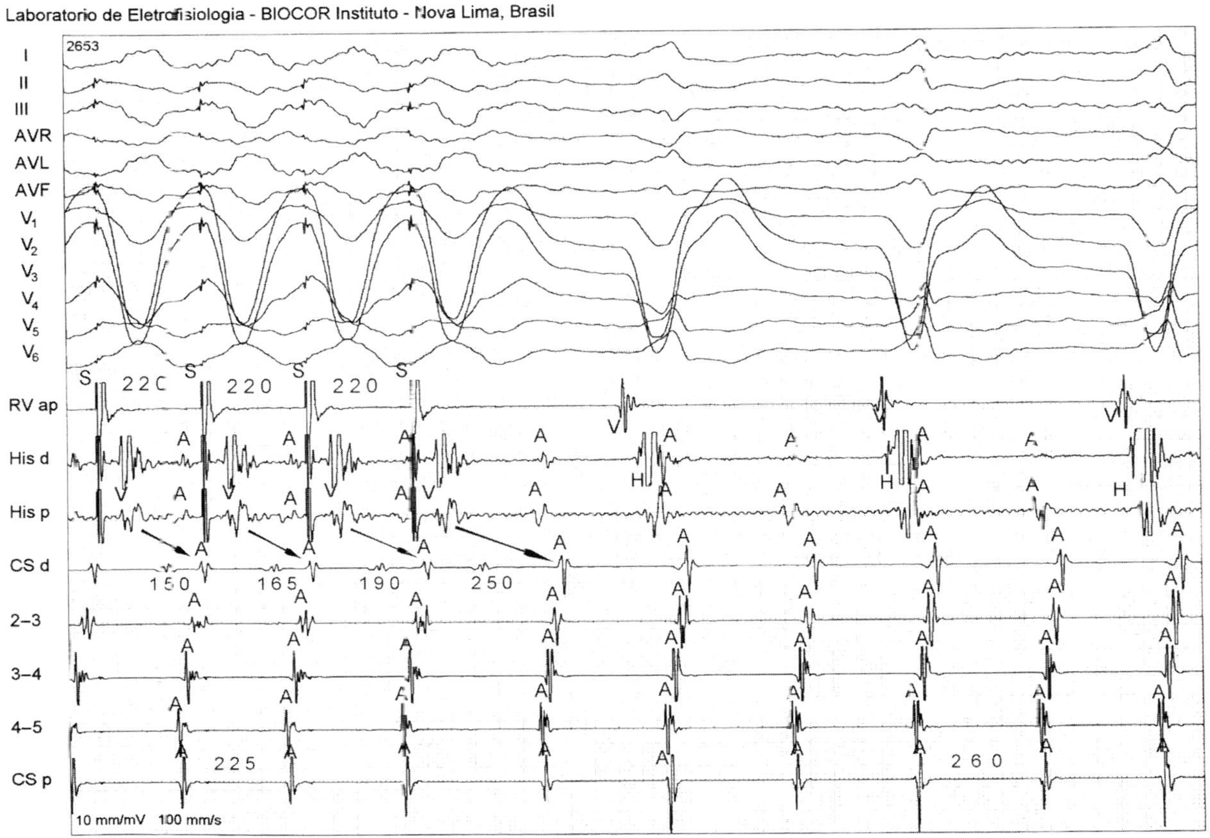

Figure 7.7 Entrainment of the tachycardia during pacing at the right ventricular apex. There was 1:1 atrial capture during ventricular pacing (cycle length 220 ms) with a similar sequence of atrial depolarization. Black arrows show decremental VA conduction through the AV node. Shown are recordings from the 12 surface ECG leads and intracardiac electrograms from the His bundle (His), right ventricular apex, and coronary sinus (CS). The recording speed was 100 mm/s.

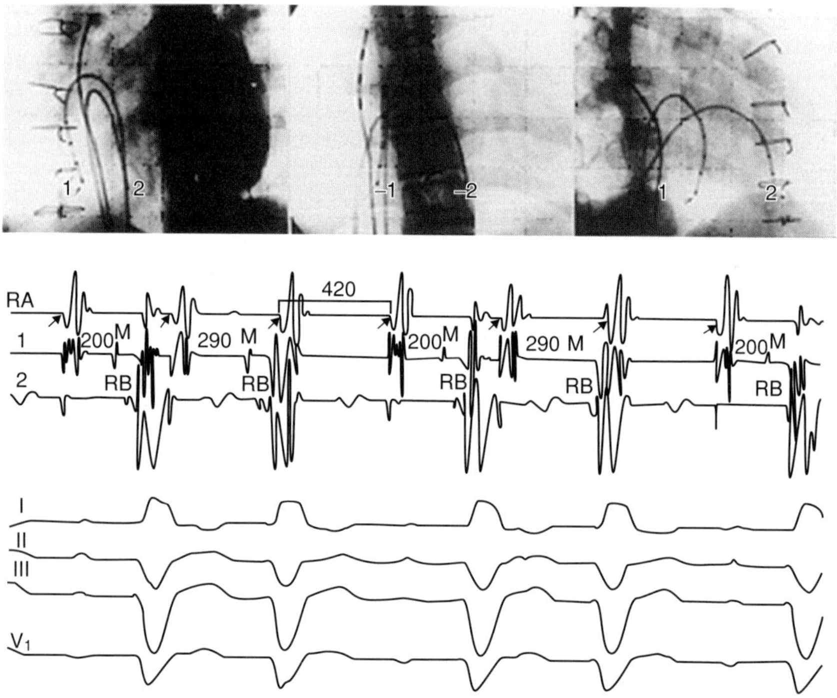

Figure 7.8 In this patient with a long AV pathway inserting in the right anteroapical region of the right ventricle (catheter 1) some distance away from catheter 2 (positioned at the distal right bundle branch in the apicoseptal region), a Wenckebach-type block occurs during right atrial pacing (RA) (at a cycle length of 420 ms). Fluoroscopy in LAO, AP, and RAO projections shows catheter 1 (at the distal insertion of the AV fiber), catheter 2 (at the distal right bundle branch), and a quadripolar catheter at the high right atrium. Sternum stitches from the previous open-heart surgery for AV node ablation are also seen. Courtesy of Dr Sosa E and Dr Scanavacca M, Heart Institute, São Paulo University, Brazil.

In our patient cohort with atriofascicular pathways, we did not find spontaneous conduction disturbances in any patient [17].

Third-degree block (spontaneous or acquired)

Normal impulse conduction through decrementally conducting fibers, in analogy with the situation with rapidly conducting accessory pathways, may disappear over the years, even after having been responsible for symptomatic tachyarrhythmias for many years. We saw two patients with atriofascicular pathways who underwent surgical AV nodal ablation as a therapeutic strategy, at a time when those fibers where supposed to be nodoventricular connections. Both patients remained preexcited, because their accessory fibers were unharmed during the surgical procedure and remained intact. No pacemaker was implanted because conduction over the accessory fiber was stable, with adequate refractoriness and an acceptable Wenckebach conduction block point. However, both patients developed syncope after six and eight years of follow-up, respectively. In both patients an electrophysiological study revealed spontaneous second-degree AV block in the decrementally conducting pathway (Fig. 7.8). Both patients received a pacemaker, and no episode of syncope occurred thereafter.

We were able to document a third-degree block in a patient with a long AV pathway who underwent radiofrequency catheter ablation [18]. The distal end of the pathway was successfully targeted, and conduction block occurred after the recording of the M potential (Figs 7.9 & 7.10).

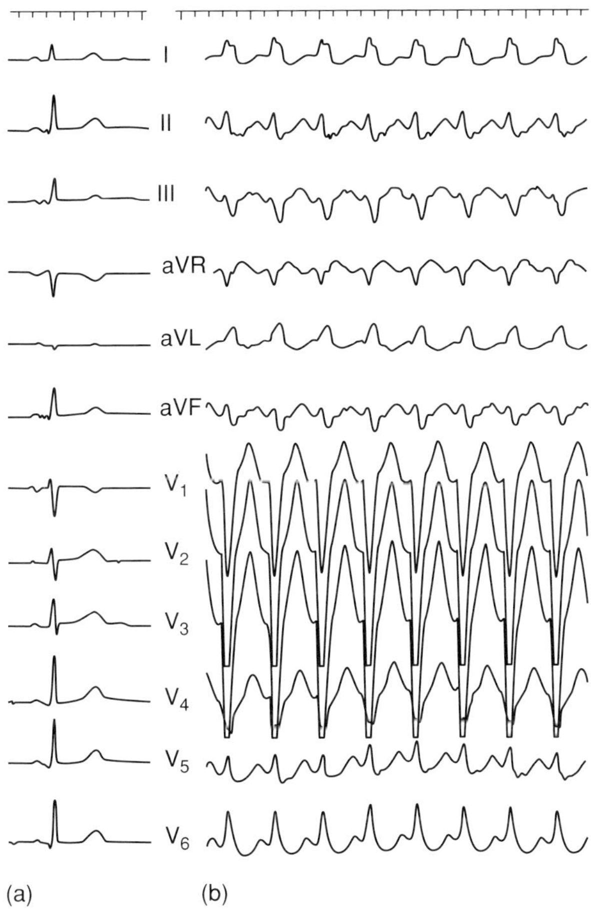

Figure 7.9 The 12-lead ECG (a) before catheter ablation and (b) during antidromic tachycardia. Paper speed: 25 mm/s.

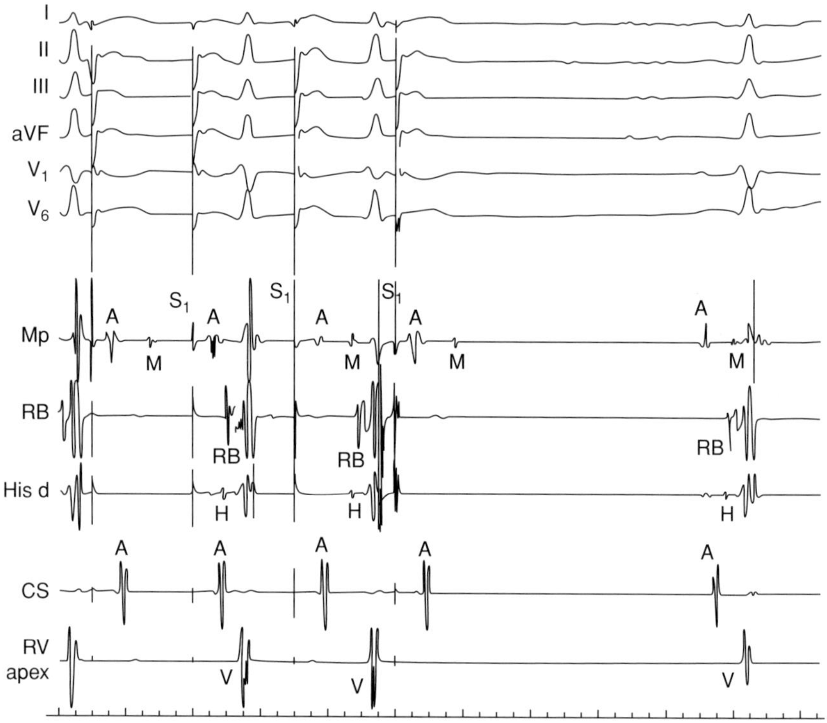

Figure 7.10 Right atrial pacing after successful catheter ablation aimed at the distal insertion of the long AV fiber. There is Wenckebach block at the AV node level with simultaneous conduction through the proximal part of the accessory fiber (AM potential interval), but complete conduction block inside this long and decrementally conducting AV pathway. Paper speed: 100 mm/s.

References

1 Davies MJ, Anderson RH, Becker AE. *The Conduction System of the Heart*. London: Butterworths; 1983.

2 Anderson RH, Ho SY. Anatomy of the atrioventricular junctions with regard to ventricular preexcitation. *PACE* 1997;20:2072.

3 Bogun F, Kalusche D, Li YG, *et al*. Septal Q waves in surface electrocardiographic lead V_6 exclude minimal ventricular preexcitation. *Am J Cardiol* 1999;84:101.

4 Lau EW, Ng GA, Griffyth MJ. A new ECG sign of an accessory pathway in sinus rhythm: pseudo partial right bundle branch block. *Heart* 1999;82:244.

5 Chen SA, Chiang CE, Tai CT, *et al*. Longitudinal clinical and electrophysiological assessment of patients with symptomatic Wolff–Parkinson–White syndrome and atrioventricular node reentrant tachycardia. *Circulation* 1996;93:2023.

6 Deal BJ, Keana JF, Gillette PC, Garson A Jr. Wolff–Parkinson–White syndrome and supraventricular tachycardia during infancy: management and follow-up. *J Am Coll Cardiol* 1985;5:130.

7 Haissaguerre M, Cauchemez B, Marcus F, *et al*. Characteristics of the ventricular insertion sites of accessory pathways with anterograde decremental conduction properties. *Circulation* 1995;91:1077.

8 Critelli G, Perticone F, Coltorti F, *et al.* Antegrade slow bypass conduction after closed-chest ablation of the His bundle in permanent junctional reciprocating tachycardia. *Circulation* 1983;67:687.
9 Sternick EB, Gerken LM, God EG. Concealed accessory pathway with long conduction times and incremental properties. A case report. *J Cardiovasc Electrophysiol* 2001;12:103.
10 Goldberger JJ, Pederson DN, Damle RS, *et al.* Antidromic tachycardia utilizing decremental, latent accessory atrioventricular fibers: differentiation from adenosine-sensitive ventricular tachycardia. *J Am Coll Cardiol* 1994;24:732.
11 Davidson NC, Morton JB, Sanders P, Kalman J. Latent Mahaim fiber as a cause of antidromic reciprocating tachycardia: recognition and successful radiofrequency ablation. *J Cardiovasc Electrophysiol* 2002;13:74.
12 Anaclerio M, Luzzi G, Forleo C, *et al.* Radiofrequency transcatheter ablation of a bidirectional decremental accessory atrioventricular pathway in the coronary sinus. *Cardiologia* 1999;44:89.
13 Peinado R, Merino JL, Ramirez L, Echeverria I. Decremental atriofascicular accessory pathway with bidirectional conduction: delineation of atrial and ventricular insertion by radiofrequency current application. *J Cardiovasc Electrophysiol* 2001;12:489.
14 Farre J, Roos D, Wiener I, *et al.* Reciprocal tachycardias using accessory pathways with long conduction times. *Am J Cardiol* 1979;44:1099.
15 Sternick EB, Fagundes M, Cruz Filho FE, *et al.* Short atrioventricular Mahaim fiber: observations on their clinical, eletrocardiographic and electrophysiologic profile. *J Cardiovasc Electrophysiol* 2005;16:127.
16 Sternick EB, Gerken LM, Scarpelli R, Wellens HJJ. Intermittent wide QRS complex during a supraventricular tachycardia. What is the mechanism? *Heart Rhythm* 2005;2.
17 Sternick EB, Timmermans C, Sosa E, *et al.* The electrocardiogram during sinus rhythm and tachycardia in patients with anterograde conduction over Mahaim fibers. The importance of an "rS" pattern in lead III. *J Am Coll Cardiol* 2004;44:1626.
18 Sternick EB, Timmermans C, Rodriguez LM, Wellens HJJ. Mahaim fiber: an atriofascicular or a long atrioventricular pathway? *Heart Rhythm* 2004;1(6):724.

CHAPTER 8

Automaticity in decrementally conducting fibers

Automatic impulse formation originates in cells with spontaneous diastolic depolarization. These cells are found in the sinus node, the atrioventricular (AV) node, the coronary sinus ostium, and the *crista terminalis*. In spite of the lack of conclusive anatomical-pathological data [1], there are strong electrophysiological arguments suggesting that decrementally conducting fibers contain accessory AV nodal tissue; some of these are as follows:

1 Slow and decremental anterograde conduction [2];

2 A structure with a proximal AV nodal component and a distal bundle branch-like component, both with His bundle-like potentials [3, 4];

3 Conduction block in response to adenosine [5];

4 Heat-induced automaticity during radiofrequency (RF) catheter ablation [6];

5 The finding of AV node-like tissue in biopsy specimens during open-heart surgery [1] in patients with atriofascicular pathways.

According to the literature, spontaneous automaticity arising in rapidly conducting accessory pathways is a very rare finding [7–9]. Spontaneous activity arising in decrementally conducting fibers has been reported [10–11]. We have studied a cohort of 40 patients with atriofascicular pathways [12] and 8 patients with short decrementally conducting AV fibers [13] to assess RF catheter ablation and spontaneously occurring cardiac arrhythmias, as well as their determinants and their clinical significance.

Since atriofascicular pathways, the most common type of decrementally conducting accessory pathways, have accessory AV nodes, we did expect to find spontaneous rhythms arising in such accessory AV nodes, in analogy with the AV node-related arrhythmias: active AV nodal rhythms and nonparoxysmal junctional tachycardia. One should also expect that automatic rhythms would be a common response of such structures when exposed to heat, as during RF catheter ablation.

Atriofascicular pathways

We retrospectively studied 40 consecutive patients with an atriofascicular or a long AV fiber in whom ablation of the accessory pathway was performed.

There were 24 females and 16 males, with a mean age of 24 ± 12 (range 8–80) years. Referral for electrophysiological assessment was based on a documented preexcited paroxysmal tachycardia, fast palpitations, or preexcited atrial fibrillation (Table 8.1). Ebstein's disease was diagnosed in 8 patients (20%). In 32

Table 8.1 Clinical data of patients with atriofascicular pathways.

Case	Sex	Age	Site	Clinical arrhythmia	*Therapy* *S/RF$_p$/RF$_d$*	*MAT* *RF$_p$*	*WPW*	*CBT*
1	F	31	L	Antidromic CMT	S			
2	F	32	L	Antidromic CMT; AVNRT	RF$_p$	Yes		
3*	F	19	PL	Antidromic CMT	RF$_p$	Yes		
4*	F	21	PL	Antidromic CMT	RF$_p$	Yes		RPS
				Ortodromic CMT	RF$_p$			
5*	M	13	PL	Antidromic CMT	RF$_p$	Yes	RPS	
6	M	52	PL	Preexcited atrial fibrillation	RF$_p$	Yes		
7*	F	19	PS	Antidromic CMT/RAS AP	RF$_p$	No	RAS	
8	F	22	P	fast palpitations	RF$_p$	Yes		
9	**M**	**21**	**L**	**Antidromic CMT**	**RF$_p$**	**Yes**		
10	F	23	L	Antidromic CMT	RF$_p$	Yes		
11	M	80	PL	AVNRT + atriofascicular bystander	RF$_p$	Yes	RPS	
12	F	19	A	Antidromic CMT	RF$_p$	Yes		
13	F	23	L	Antidromic CMT	RF$_p$	Yes		
14	F	25	PL	Antidromic CMT	RF$_p$	Yes		
15	M	35	L	Antidromic CMT	RF$_p$	Yes		
16	F	42	L	Antidromic CMT	RF$_p$	Yes		
17	F	23	L	Antidromic CMT	RF$_p$	Yes		
18	**F**	**8**	**AL**	**Atriofascicular automaticity**	**RF$_p$**	**Yes**		
19	M	30	PL	Antidromic CMT	RF$_p$	Yes		
20	F	27	L	Antidromic CMT	RF$_p$	Yes		
21	F	19	L	Antidromic CMT	RF$_p$	Yes		
22	**M**	**12**	**MS**	**Atriofascicular automaticity**	**RF$_p$**	**No**		
23	F	39	L	Antidromic CMT	RF$_p$	Yes		
24*	F	12	L	Antidromic CMT	RF$_p$	No	RL	
25	F	15	AL	AVNRT + atriofascicular bystander	RF$_p$	Yes		
26	M	13	L	Antidromic CMT	RF$_p$	Yes		
27	M	15	A	Antidromic CMT	RF$_p$	Yes		
28	F	25	L	Antidromic CMT	RF$_p$	Yes		
29*	M	17	L	Antidromic CMT	RF$_p$	Yes	RPS	RL
				Ortodromic CMT				
30	M	18	L	Antidromic CMT	RF$_p$	Yes		
31	F	45	L	Antidromic CMT	RF$_p$	Yes		
32	M	24	L	Antidromic CMT	RF$_d$			
33*	**M**	**11**	**L**	**Antidromic CMT**	**S**			
34*	M	26	L	Antidromic CMT	RF$_d$			LL
35	M	25	A	Antidromic CMT	RF$_d$			
36	**F**	**26**	**P**	**Antidromic CMT**	**RF$_d$**			
37	F	31	L	Antidromic CMT	RF$_d$			
38	F	22	L	Antidromic CMT; AVNRT	RF$_p$	Yes		
39	F	17	L	Antidromic CMT	RF$_p$	Yes		
40	M	17	P	Antidromic CMT	RF$_p$	Yes		

Note: Bold indicates patients with spontaneous automaticity.

*Patient with Ebstein's disease.

Antidromic CMT, antidromic circus movement tachycardia with anterograde conduction over the atriofascicular fiber; CBT, concealed bypass tract; MAT, Mahaim automatic tachycardia during RF ablation; RAS, right anteroseptal accessory pathway; S, surgical ablation; RFp, radiofrequency catheter ablation targeting proximal Mahaim potential at the annulus; RFd, radiofrequency ablation targeting distal insertion. The site was tricuspid annulus (A, anterior; AL, anterolateral; L, lateral; MS, midseptal; P, posterior; PL, posterolateral; PS, posteroseptal).

patients the atrial insertion of the fiber was identified by localizing a discrete accessory pathway potential, and in 8 patients by assessing the shortest AV interval during atrial pacing at different sites. All patients underwent successful surgical ($n = 2$) or RF catheter ablation ($n = 38$). In 32 patients RF ablation was done from the atrial end, and in 6 patients it was done from the ventricular end after right ventricular pacemapping. Five patients (cases 9, 18, 22, 33, and 36) showed spontaneous automaticity (Table 8.1).

Spontaneous automaticity

The 5 patients with spontaneous automaticity were younger than the 35 patients without spontaneous automaticity (15 ± 7 vs. 26 ± 13 years), but the difference did not reach statistical significance ($p = 0.09$). Three were male, with one having Ebstein's disease. None of the 5 patients had an associated rapidly conducting accessory AV pathway (AP). Although the number of patients is too small for comparison, clinical presentation of patients with antidromic tachycardia did not differ from that of atriofascicular patients without spontaneous automaticity. In the 5 patients (12.5%) spontaneous automatic rhythms were found with the same QRS complex configuration as during maximal preexcitation automaticity rates ranged from a slow rhythm occurring during the night, indistinguishable from an accelerated idioventricular rhythm (AIVR) with a cycle length of 900 ms, to nonsustained repetitive tachycardia with a cycle length of 360 ms (Table 8.2). Three patients were referred because an antidromic tachycardia with anterograde conduction over the atriofascicular fiber also showed spontaneous automaticity. QRS complex configuration was identical during the reentrant and the automatic rhythm (Fig. 8.1). In one patient (case 36), episodes of asymptomatic slow automatic rhythm resembling AIVR occurred at a slower rate during the nighttime and at a faster rate during daytime (Fig. 8.2). In two patients (cases 18 and 22), automaticity was the clinical problem. They sought medical treatment because of a long history

Table 8.2 Electrophysiological data of patients with an atriofascicular pathway and spontaneous automaticity.

n	*Case*	*Clinical arrhythmia*	*AM CL range (ms)*	*Diagnosis by*	*Isuprel Acceleration*	*VA conduction atriofascicular AV node*	*MAT*
1	18	automatic runs	550–450	ECG	*	no / no	yes
2	22	automatic runs	360–400	ECG	*	no / yes	no
3	9	a-CMT	720–580	EPS	***	no / yes	yes
4	33	a-CMT	840–550	Holter*/EPS	***	no / yes	
5	36	a-CMT	900–530	Holter*/EPS	**	no / yes	

*Before EPS automatic rhythms were diagnosed as AIVR.
a-CMT, antidromic circus movement tachycardia; AM, automaticity in atriofascicular fiber; CL, cycle length; MAT, Mahaim automatic tachycardia during radiofrequency ablation of the atrial insertion; EPS, electrophysiological study.

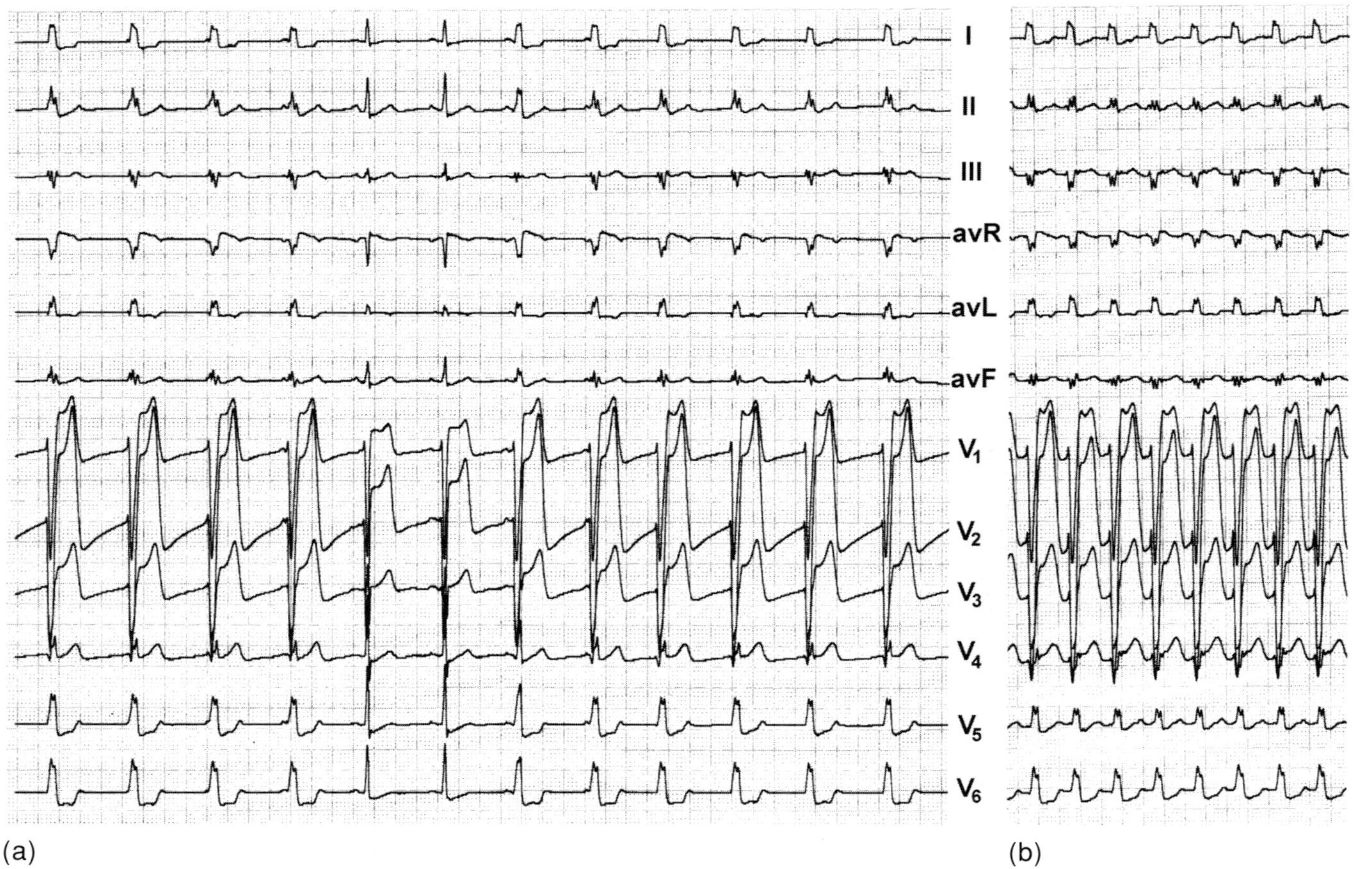

Figure 8.1 Spontaneous atriofascicular automatic rhythm (a) and antidromic tachycardia showing the same QRS complex morphology (b).

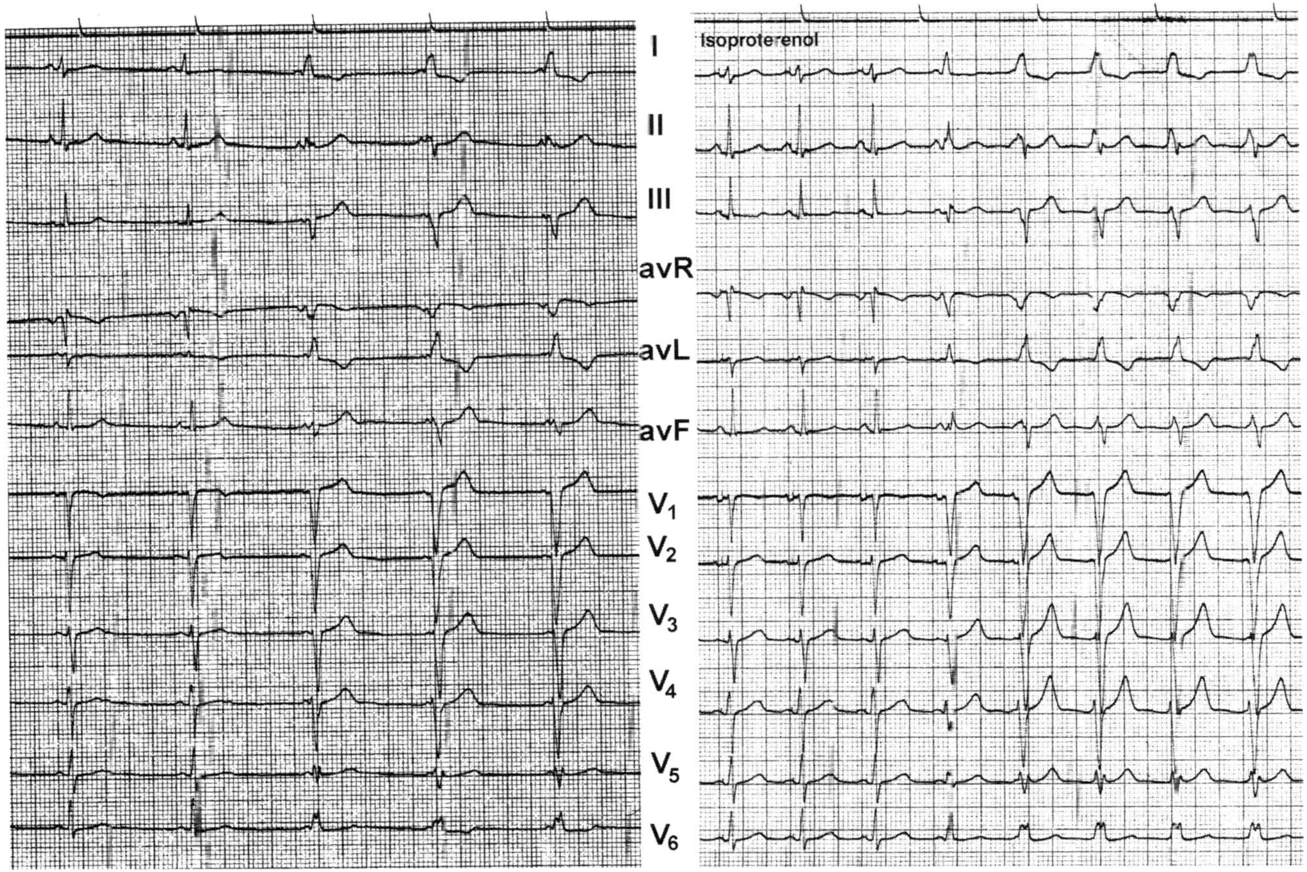

Figure 8.2 Case 36:(a) 12-lead ECG showing sinus rhythm and Mahaim automaticity at 60 beats/min (third QRS complex is a fusion beat); (b) during isoproterenol infusion both sinus rhythm (580 ms) and Mahaim automaticity (640 ms) accelerate (fourth QRS complex is a fusion beat).

of repetitive fast palpitations. Both showed repetitive bursts of nonsustained tachycardia with a left bundle branch block (LBBB)-like configuration.

There was ventriculoatrial (VA) dissociation during the majority of the episodes, but in case 18 some tachycardias showed 2:1 retrograde VA conduction over the AV node. In patients showing automaticity, the automatic rhythm was recorded during the electrophysiological study before the administration of isoproterenol. During isoproterenol infusion there was an increase in both the rate and the duration of the episodes. This effect was less pronounced in the two patients with repetitive nonsustained automatic runs. They showed only a slight increase in automaticity rate. Electrophysiological validation of the site of origin of this automatic rhythm included the recording of an M potential preceding the preexcited QRS complex and retrograde depolarization of the right bundle followed by the His bundle. In patient 9 (Fig. 8.3), there was VA dissociation during the automatic rhythm.

During atrial overdrive stimulation there was a transient suppression without entrainment, acceleration, or persistent termination of the tachycardia in cases 18 and 22. Following stimulation, tachycardia resumed almost immediately in cases 18 and 22.

Induction of antidromic CMT by the automatic rhythm

In two patients (cases 9 and 33) the automatic rhythm triggered episodes of antidromic tachycardia (Fig. 8.4). In both cases it happened during isoproterenol infusion. Initiation of antidromic tachycardia was preceded by a long RR cycle due to AV dissociation caused by automatic beats arising in the atriofascicular fiber. The preceding P wave, which was not conducted through the AV node, was conducted with critical slowing in the fiber (Fig. 8.4). Isoproterenol improved retrograde conduction over the AV node, enabling antidromic circus movement tachycardia to become sustained, but the mode of tachycardia induction was not related to the VA conduction itself or to the slowing of the sinus rate.

Heat-induced automaticity

Automaticity occurred at the proximal insertion of the atriofascicular fiber: Mahaim automatic tachycardia (MAT) was induced during RF catheter ablation in 30 out of 33 patients (91%) when ablation was targeted at the proximal Mahaim potential at the atrial aspect of the tricuspid annulus. MAT usually started promptly after current delivery (usually in less than 5 s). The MAT duration was variable, lasting from 4 beats to almost 2 min (Fig. 8.5). Its occurrence could not be prevented by atrial pacing during catheter ablation. In 4 patients with prolonged MAT, successful ablation was only achieved after complete elimination of this rhythm (Fig. 8.5b).

Automaticity during ablation at the distal insertion of the atriofascicular fiber

We did not include in these results the 5 patients who were ablated targeting the distal insertion (Table 8.1). They did develop automaticity, but because

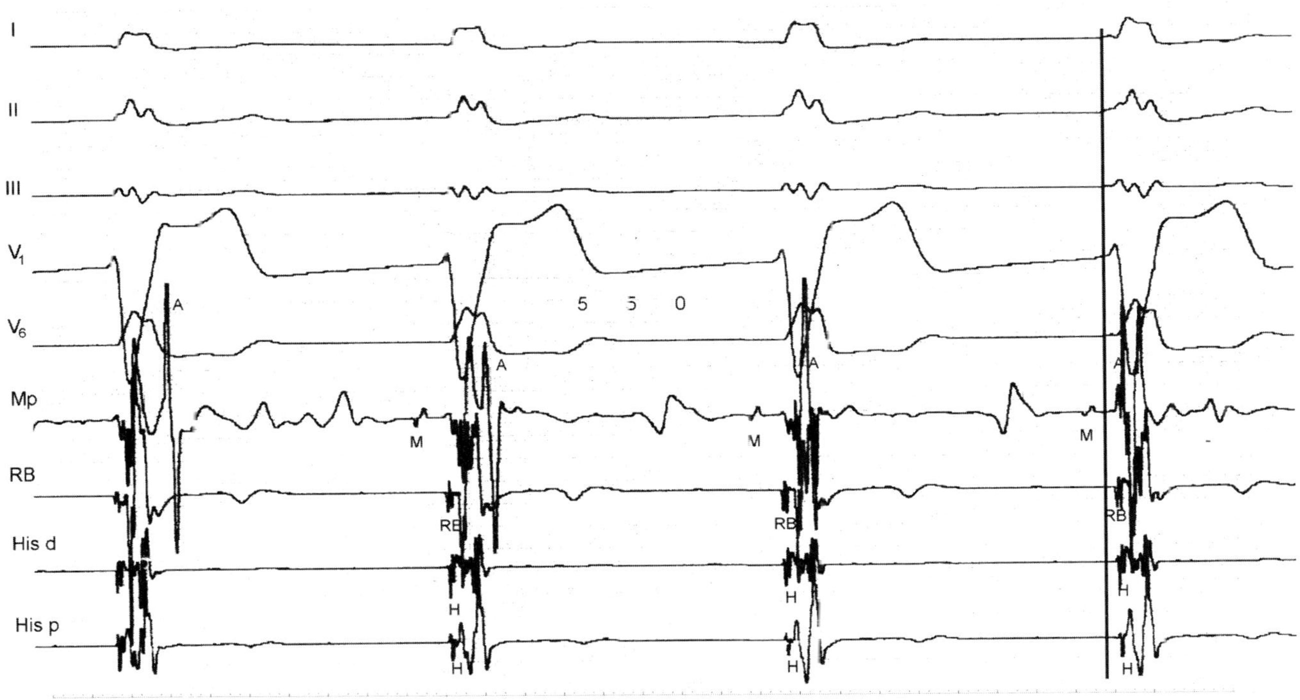

Figure 8.3 Case 9: registration during the electrophysiological study at 100 mm/s showing an automatic rhythm with LBBB-like morphology. A Mahaim (M) potential precedes each QRS (MV interval = 50 ms). There is retrograde activation of the distal conduction system (right bundle followed by the His bundle potential) but without retrograde conduction to the atrial level, where the rhythm is clearly dissociated from that in the ventricle.

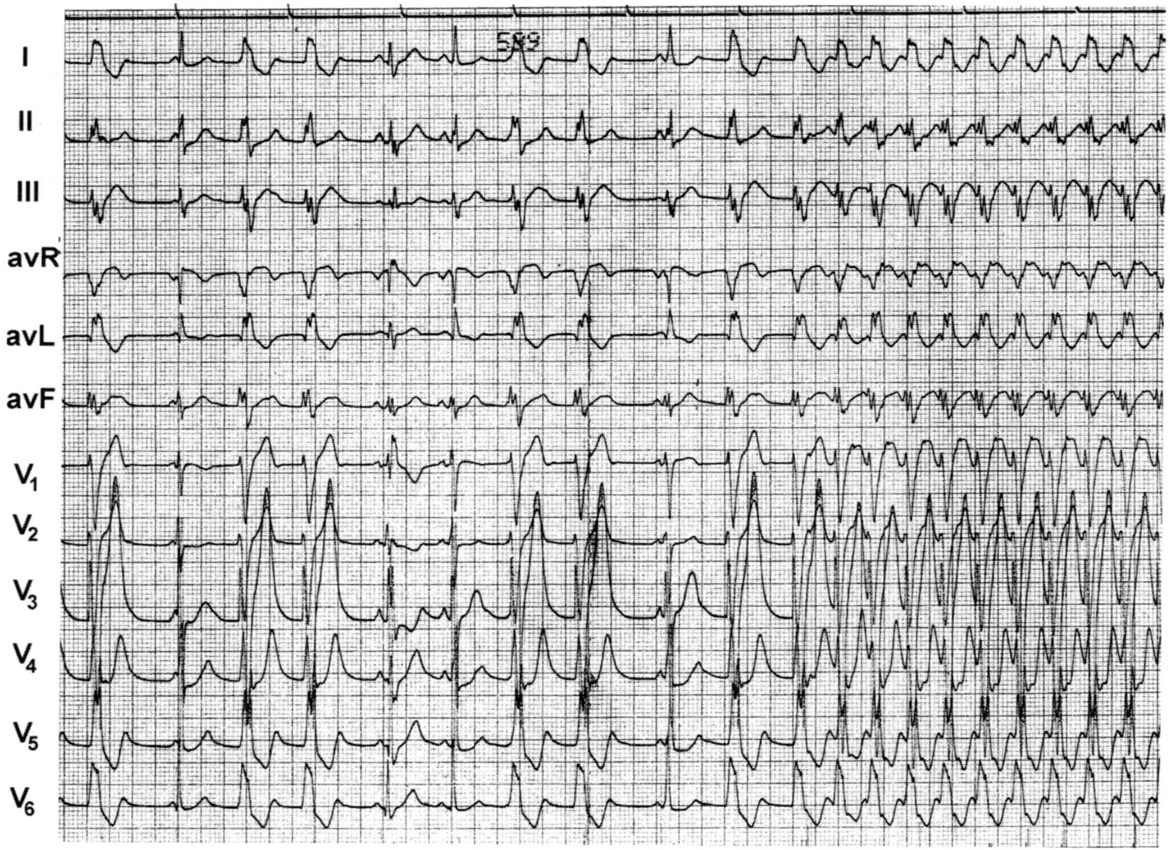

Figure 8.4 Case 33: 12-lead ECG showing automatic beats among minimally preexcited sinus beats. Antidromic circus movement tachycardia is triggered by an automatic beat with retrograde VA conduction through the AV node.

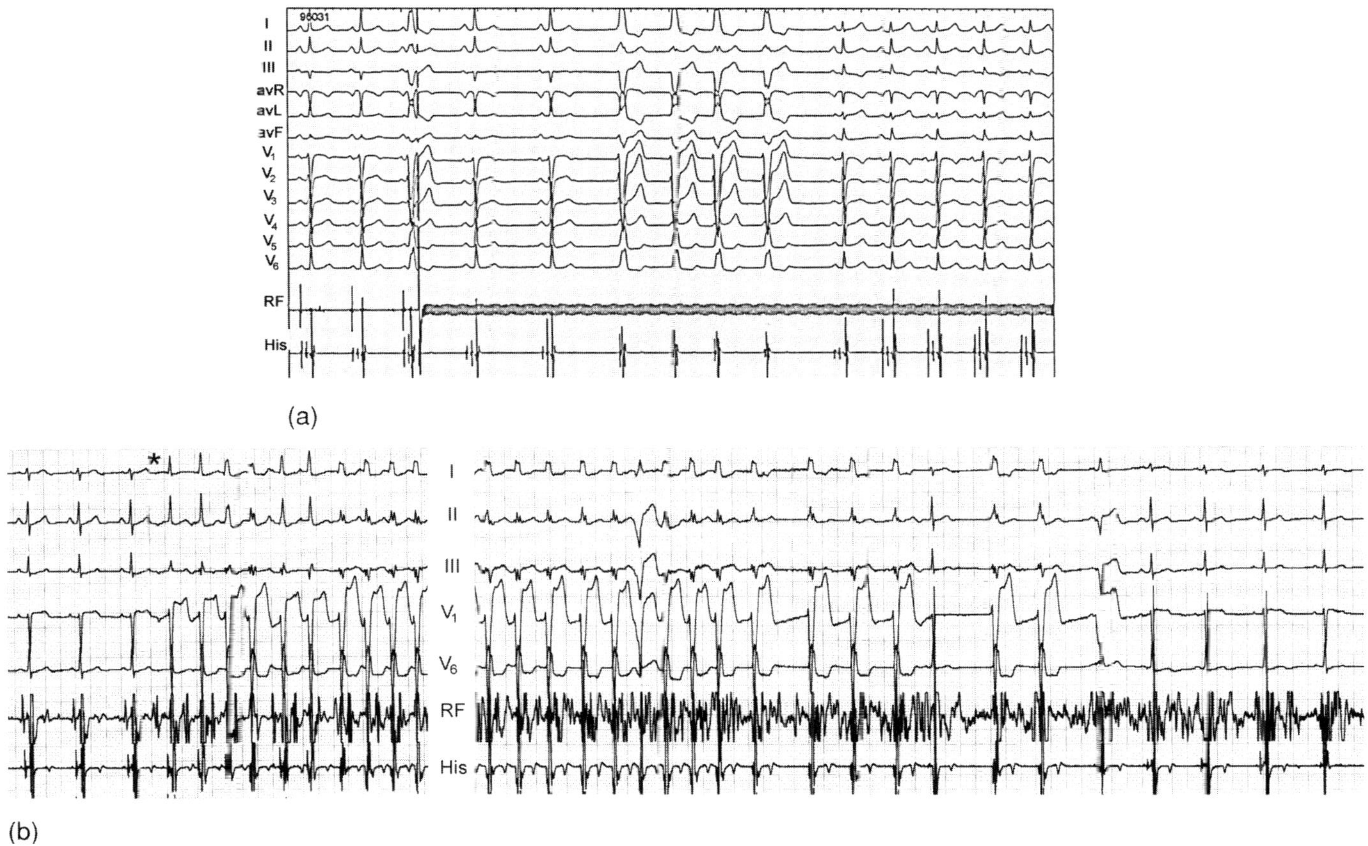

Figure 8.5 (a) A short episode of atriofascicular automaticity consisting of 4 beats with LBBB-like morphology. Minimal ventricular preexcitation is present before (see rS pattern in lead III) and absent thereafter (qR in lead III). (b) Mahaim automaticity starts immediately after RF current delivery (*), lasting almost 1 min. After MAT was completely terminated, Mahaim conduction did not recur.

there were slight differences in QRS configuration, we could not rule out that the rhythm was arising in the distal part of the right bundle branch or in the ventricular myocardium. Early investigators [1, 3, 4, 14, 15] suggested that Mahaim fibers could be a complete accessory AV conduction pathway with variable length containing AV node-like tissue. Intracardiac electrophysiological evaluation has been the main tool to solve the Mahaim puzzle. Transient accelerated automatic rhythms arising from the Mahaim fiber during RF catheter ablation [6, 16, 17] have been recognized as one of the features that such fibers share with AV nodal tissue. These rhythms are analogous to the accelerated junctional rhythm (AJR) arising during slow AV nodal pathway ablation in patients with AV node reentrant tachycardia (AVNRT). AJR is considered to be a sensitive marker [18] of a successful ablation site. It seems that heat-induced automaticity is as common during ablation of Mahaim fibers as during slow AV nodal pathway ablation. We found it in 30 out of 33 patients (91%) when the atrial insertion was targeted. Other authors reported similar figures: for example, Braun *et al.* [17] found it in 100% of the patients (15 out of 15 cases), while Heald *et al.* [16] found it in 57% (12 out of 21 cases).

We found in 4 patients that complete termination of heat-induced automaticity may be required as an ablation endpoint to achieve long-term success [6].

Spontaneous automaticity arising in a Mahaim fiber was first reported by Kanter *et al.* [19] in a 7-year-old child with incessant bigeminy, initially thought to be of ventricular origin. She underwent electrophysiological evaluation because a 24-hour Holter monitoring showed nonsustained runs suggestive of ventricular tachycardia. During the electrophysiological study an atriofascicular pathway was diagnosed. Sosa and Scanavacca [10] reported a patient with symptomatic runs of an irregular LBBB-like tachycardia with AV dissociation, which was most likely due to spontaneous automaticity. Belhassen *et al.* [11] reported one patient with a likely automatic escape rhythm arising in an atriofascicular pathway. It is remarkable to find spontaneous automaticity in 12.5% of our large cohort of 40 patients with atriofascicular fibers. These young patients presented with a spectrum of automatic rhythms, ranging from asymptomatic slow rhythms to fast and repetitive bursts of tachycardia with LBBB-like morphology. They share these findings with patients having AV nodal automaticity [20]. There are a few reports [21–23] about young patients with AVNRT showing spontaneous AJR, which can be cured by slow pathway modification with RF catheter ablation. Epstein *et al.* [23] found in 3 out of 5 patients that AJR served as trigger for AVNRT, particularly with AJR at an accelerated rate. Our observation was the same in 2 of 5 patients who had antidromic CMT triggered by automatic beats. Epstein *et al.* [23] reported a 17% incidence (5 out of 29 patients) of spontaneous episodic AJR in a population with a mean age of 12.9 ± 5.2 (range 4.2–25) years, which is similar to that in our study population with a mean age of 15 ± 7 (8–26) years. We also found that spontaneous automaticity was terminated after successful catheter ablation; this matched the observation of Epstein *et al.* [23] that in their patients with AJR and AVNRT it was required to eliminate or drastically modulate the AJR to achieve a long-term successful result.

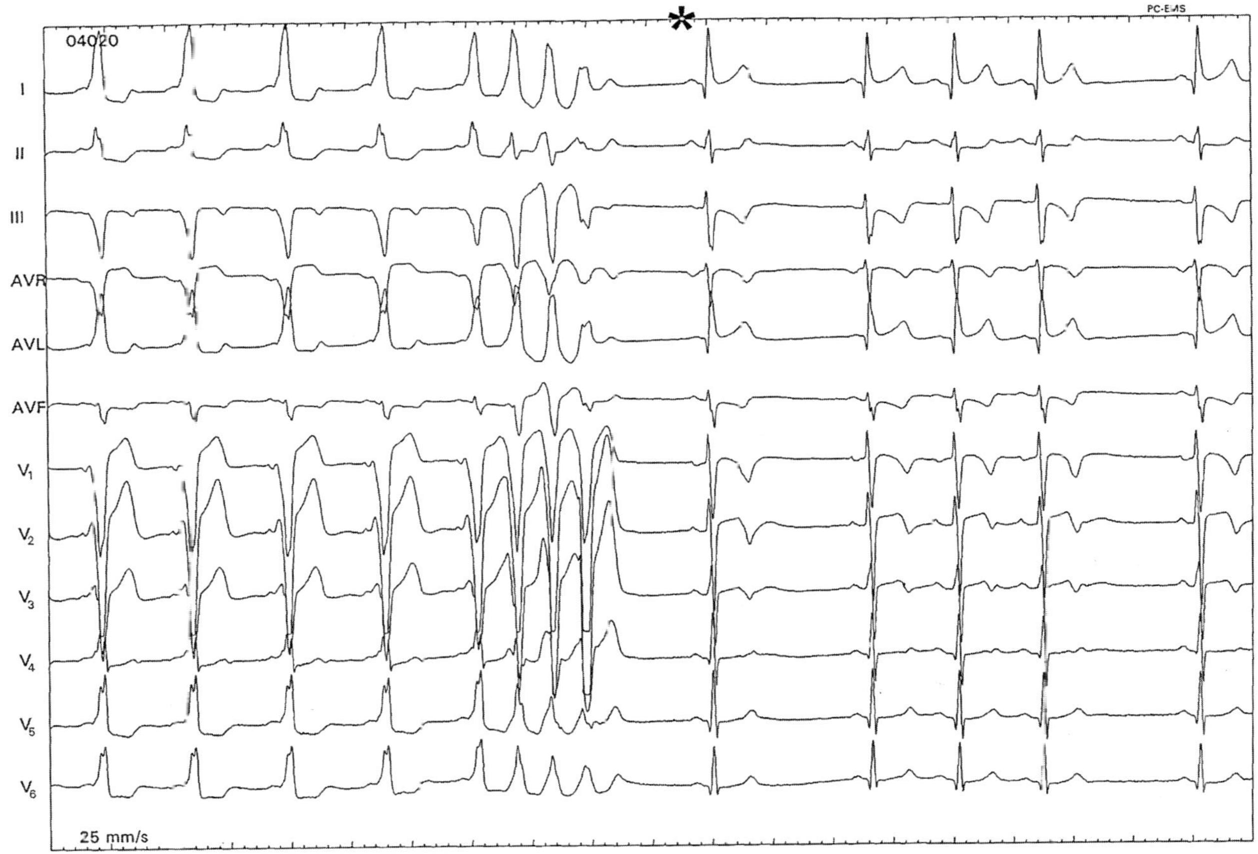

Figure 8.6 A short run of heat-induced automatic rhythm in a patient with a short AV decrementally conducting fiber occurring just before permanent block during RF catheter ablation.

The likely mechanism of spontaneous rhythms as seen in cases 9, 33, and 36 was normal automaticity. In these patients, Mahaim automaticity was dependent on the slowing of the sinus rate ("Mahaim escape rhythm") (Fig. 8.2). Isoproterenol infusion increased both sinus and Mahaim automaticity, but in these patients a greater increase in the discharge rate was seen at the Mahaim fiber level ("Mahaim active rhythm"). Patients 18 and 22 had an incessant repetitive nonsustained tachycardia that could neither be terminated nor be induced by programmed electrical stimulation. Isoproterenol infusion in these patients caused only a slight increase in the discharge rate. These findings also suggest abnormal automaticity as the mechanism of their clinical tachycardia.

Short AV decrementally conducting fibers

In a cohort of 8 patients with a short AV decrementally conducting fiber, no spontaneous automatic rhythm was found during the 24-hour ambulatory Holter monitoring or during electrophysiological study [13]. However, in 4 patients, short-lived automaticity was brought about during RF catheter ablation (Fig. 8.6). Automaticity in these patients heralded successful ablation in much the same way as in patients with atriofascicular pathways. In 3 of the 4 patients who developed RF-induced automaticity, intravenous adenosine infused before ablation caused transient conduction block in the decremental pathway. In at least 50% of the patients in this small cohort of those with decrementally conducting accessory pathways, we found electrophysiological evidence suggestive of an AV node-like structure, although it lacked the long branching portion like the one occurring in atriofascicular or long AV fibers.

Conclusion

Mahaim fiber automaticity occurring during catheter ablation of its atrial insertion is a very common event, occurring in more than 90% of patients, and its complete termination may be required in some patients to achieve long-term success. Short- lived heat-induced automaticity may also occur in some patients having short decrementally conducting AV fibers.

Spontaneous automaticity arising in the Mahaim fiber was observed only in atriofascicular pathways. It can be a trigger for antidromic circus movement tachycardia, and in some instances it can be a major clinical problem. Automaticity in Mahaim fibers is another characteristic that it shares with the electrophysiological behavior of the AV node.

References

1 Guiraudon CM, Guiraudon GM, Klein GJ. Histologic evidence for an accessory atrioventricular pathway with AV-node like morphology. *Circulation* 1988;78(suppl 2):40.

2 Wellens HJJ. *Electrical Stimulation of the Heart in the Study and Treatment of Tachycardias.* Baltimore: University Park Press; 1971.

3 Klein GJ, Guiraudon GM, Kerr CR, *et al.* "Nodoventricular" accessory pathway: evidence for a distinct accessory atrioventricular pathway with atrioventricular node-like properties. *J Am Coll Cardiol* 1988;11:1035.

4 McClelland JH, Wang X, Beckman KJ, *et al.* Radiofrequency catheter ablation of right atriofascicular (Mahaim) accessory pathways guided by accessory pathway activation potentials. *Circulation* 1994;89:2655.

5 Ellenbogen KA, Rogers R, Old W. Pharmacological characterization of conduction over a Mahaim fiber: evidence for adenosine sensitive conduction. *Pacing Clin Electrophysiol* 1989;12:1396.

6 Sternick EB, Gerken LM, Vrandecic MO. Appraisal of "Mahaim" automatic tachycardia. *J Cardiovasc Electrophysiol* 2002;13:244.

7 Macle L, Shah DC, Jais P, Haissaguerre M. Accessory pathway automaticity after radiofrequency ablation. *J Cardiovasc Electrophysiol* 2002;13:285.

8 Lerman BB, Josephson ME. Automaticity of the Kent bundle: confirmation by phase 3 and phase 4 block. *J Am Coll Cardiol* 1985;5:996.

9 Tseng ZH, Yadav AV, Scheinman MM. Catecholamine dependent accessory pathway automaticity. *Pacing Clin Electrophysiol* 2004;27:1005.

10 Sosa E, Scanavacca M. Repetitive, non-sustained wide QRS complex tachycardia: what is the tachycardia mechanism? *J Cardiovasc Electrophysiol* 2001;12:977.

11 Belhassen B, Ilan M, Glick A. Wide QRS rhythm in a young woman with recurrent palpitations: what is the diagnosis? *J Cardiovasc Electrophysiol* 2003;14:1376.

12 Sternick EB, Timmermans C, Sosa E, *et al.* Automaticity in Mahaim fibers. *J Cardiovasc Electrophysiol* 2004;15:738.

13 Sternick EB, Fagundes M, Cruz Filho FE, *et al.* Short atrioventricular Mahaim Fiber: observations on their clinical, eletrocardiographic and electrophysiologic profile. *J Cardiovasc Electrophysiol* 2005;16:127.

14 Haissaguerre M, Cauchemez B, Marcus F, *et al.* Characteristics of the ventricular insertion sites of accessory pathways with anterograde decremental conduction properties. *Circulation* 1995;91:1077.

15 Kuck KH, Siebels J, Braun E, *et al.* Mahaim fibers – a second atrioventricular conduction system. *Pacing Clin Electrophysiol* 1997;20:1201.

16 Heald SC, Davies W, Ward DE, *et al.* Radiofrequency catheter ablation of Mahaim tachycardia by targeting Mahaim potentials at the tricuspid annulus. *Br Heart J* 1995;73:250.

17 Braun E, Siebbels J, Volkmer M, *et al.* Radiofrequency-induced preexcited automatic rhythm during ablation accessory pathways with Mahaim-type preexcitation: does it predict clinical outcome? *Pacing Clin Electrophysiol* 1997;20:1121.

18 Thakur RR, Klein GJ, Yee R. Junctional tachycardia: a useful marker during radiofrequency ablation for atrioventricular node reentrant tachycardia. *J Am Coll Cardiol* 1993;22:1706.

19 Kanter R, Saba Z, Garson A Jr. Wide complex bigeminy: unusual presentation of an atriofascicular fiber. *J Cardiovasc Electrophysiol* 1994;5:795.

20 Lee PC, Kanter R, Gomez-Marin O, *et al.* Quantitative assessment of the recovery property of atriofascicular/atrioventricular-type Mahaim fiber. *J Cardiovasc Electrophysiol* 2002;13:535.

21 Ehlert FA, Goldberger JJ, Deal BJ, *et al.* Successful radiofrequency energy ablation of automatic junctional tachycardia preserving normal atrio-ventricular nodal conduction. *Pacing Clin Electrophysiol* 1993;16:54.

22 Levy AM, Bonazinga BJ. Sudden sinus slowing with junctional escape: a common mode of initiation of juvenile supraventricular tachycardia. *Circulation* 1983;67:84.

23 Epstein MR, Saul JP, Fishberger SB, *et al*. Spontaneous accelerated junctional rhythm: an unusual but useful observation prior to radiofrequency catheter ablation for atrioventricular node reentrant tachycardia in young patients. *Pacing Clin Electrophysiol* 1997; 20:1654.

CHAPTER 9

Differential diagnosis of left bundle branch block-shaped tachycardias

Introduction

The correct diagnosis of the site of origin of a regular tachycardia with a wide QRS complex (>120 ms) is important for management and prognosis of patients. Over the last 40 years, a number of approaches have been suggested to help a physician in this challenging decision making [1–14]. Intravenous medications, particularly verapamil or diltiazem, erroneously given because of a misdiagnosis of supraventricular tachycardia (SVT) can be deleterious because they may precipitate hemodynamic collapse in a patient with ventricular tachycardia (VT). Stable vital signs during tachycardia are not helpful for distinguishing SVT from VT. If the diagnosis of SVT cannot be proven or made easily, then the patient should be treated as if VT were present [15]. The focus should be on the electrocardiogram (ECG) signs, which may not only help to distinguish between a VT and other tachycardias with a broad QRS complex but also suggest its etiology and site of origin in the ventricle.

Classification of left bundle branch block-shaped tachycardias

Left bundle branch block (LBBB)-shaped (LBBB) tachycardias can be divided into three groups (Fig. 9.1).

1 SVT with preexistent or functional LBBB:
  (a) preexistent LBBB;
  (b) tachycardia-dependent phase 3 block;
  (c) retrograde invasion into the LBB;
  (d) LBBB induced by drugs (pseudo VT).

2 SVT with atrioventricular (AV) conduction over a right-sided accessory pathway:
  (a) rapidly conducting accessory pathways;
  (b) slowly conducting accessory (Mahaim) pathways.

3 Monomorphic VT:
  (a) ectopic ventricular origin;
  (b) bundle branch reentry

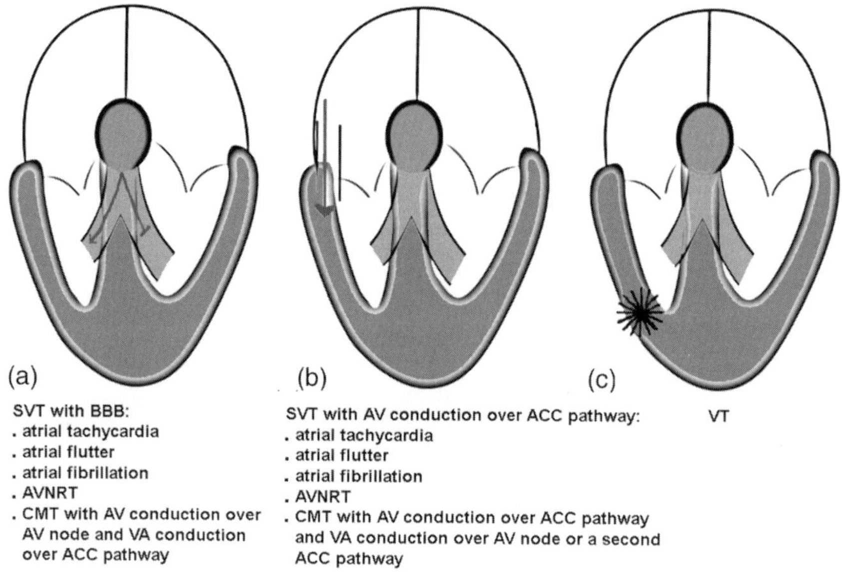

Figure 9.1 (a) Different types of SVT with LBBB, (b) SVT with AV conduction over an accessory pathway, and (c), VT resulting in a broad QRS complex tachycardia.
Acc, accessory; AV, atrioventricular; BBB, bundle branch block; CMT, circus movement tachycardia; SVT, supraventricular tachycardia; VA, ventriculoatrial; VT, ventricular tachycardia.

The ECG diagnosis

AV dissociation

Although dissociation between atrial and ventricular activity during tachycardia is a hallmark of VT (lead II, Fig. 9.2), some form of VA conduction may be present during VT, particularly during a slow VT (Fig. 9.3) [7]. P waves can be difficult to recognize during a broad QRS tachycardia, and it can be useful to look for nonelectrocardiographic signs such as variations in jugular pulsations, the loudness of the first heart sound, and changes in systolic blood pressure [16]. In patients with slow VT rates, occasional conduction from atrium to ventricle over the AV node bundle branch system may happen resulting in "capture" or "fusion" beats.

Sudden narrowing of a QRS complex during VT may also be the result of a premature ventricular depolarization arising in the ventricle in which the tachycardia originates, or it may occur when retrograde conduction during VT produces a ventricular echo beat leading to fusion with the VT QRS complex. Very rarely AV dissociation is present in tachycardias other than VT. It may occur in AV junctional tachycardia (JET) after cardiac surgery or during digitalis intoxication. AV dissociation has been reported during narrow QRS complex tachycardia due to nodofascicular (NF) fibers either manifest or concealed [17, 18].

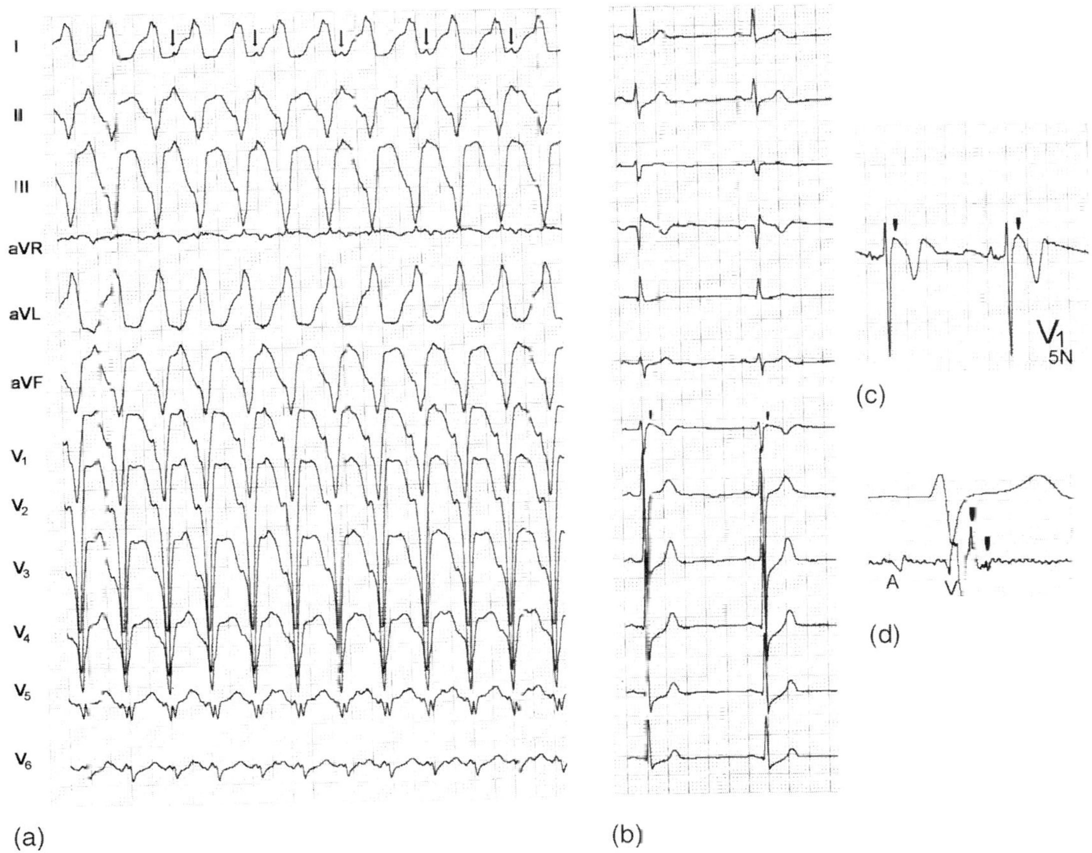

Figure 9.2 (a) LBBB-shaped VT in a patient with arrhythmogenic right ventricular dysplasia (ARVD) with AV dissociation (arrow points to P waves). (b) Black arrowhead in V1 during sinus rhythm, points to epsilom wave, which can be better seen in (c), (d) shows a late potential in the corresponding intracavitary recording.

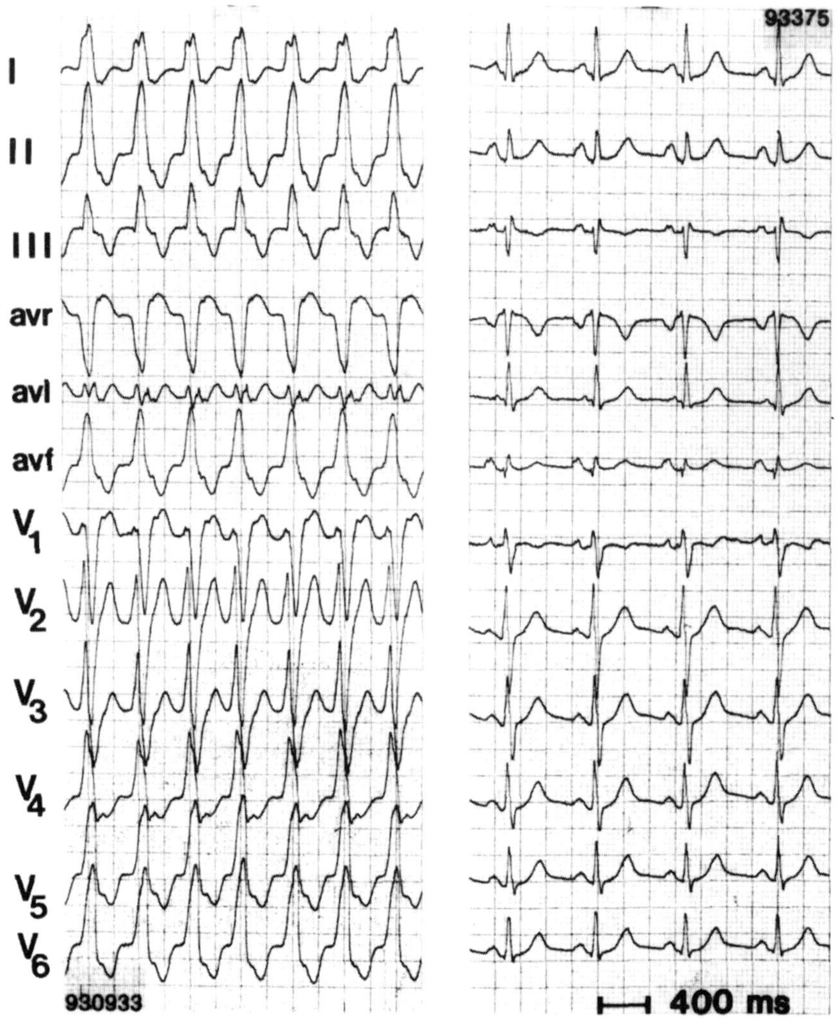

(a) (b)

Figure 9.3 (a) One-to-one VA conduction during an idiopathic VT from the inflow tract of the right ventricle. The P waves are negative in the inferior leads and follow each QRS complex. (b) The same patient during sinus rhythm.

Width of the QRS complex

As pointed out by Wellens [19], and shown in Fig. 9.4, the site of origin of VT plays a role in the width of the QRS complex. When the arrhythmia arises far from the interventricular septum, the sequential activation of the ventricles results in a very wide QRS.

The QRS complex will be narrower when VT has its origin in or close to the septum. Other factors, such as the size of the scar tissue (after myocardial

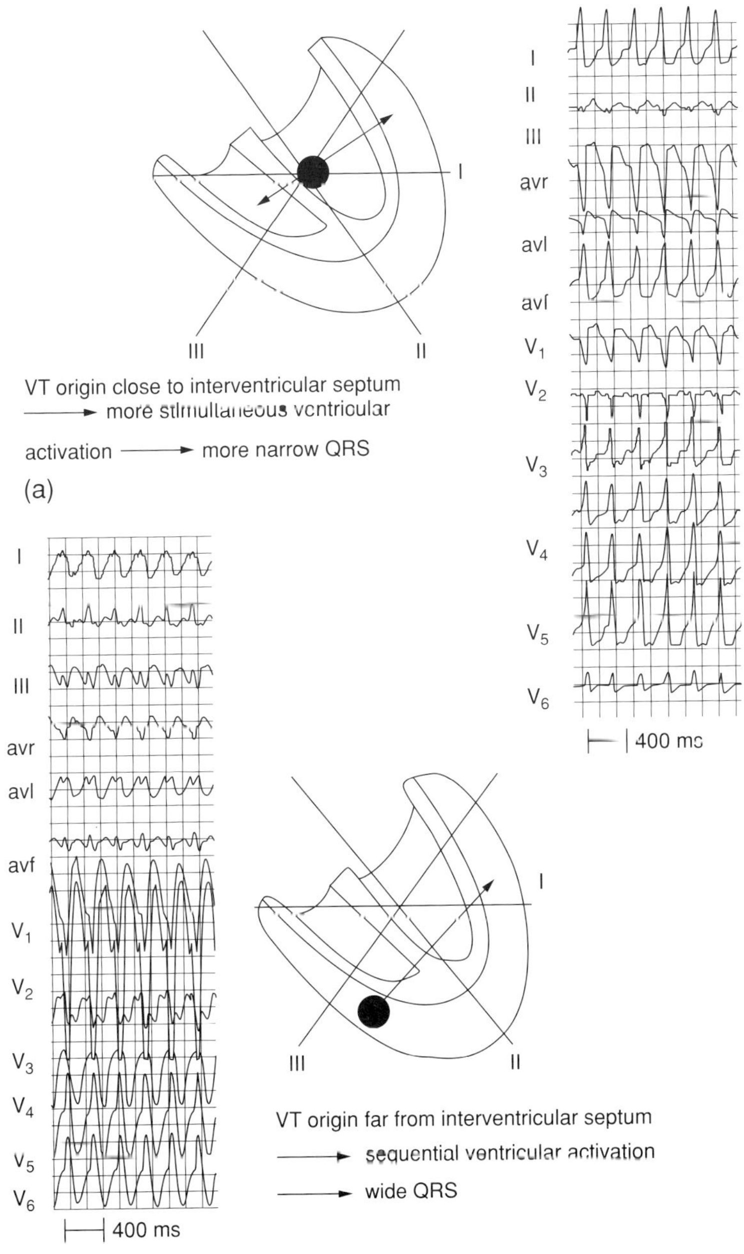

Figure 9.4 VT origin and QRS width. (a) An origin close to the interventricular septum results in more simultaneous right and left ventricular activation and therefore a narrower QRS complex. (b) In contrast, a VT origin in the right ventricular free wall results in sequential ventricular activation and a wider QRS complex.

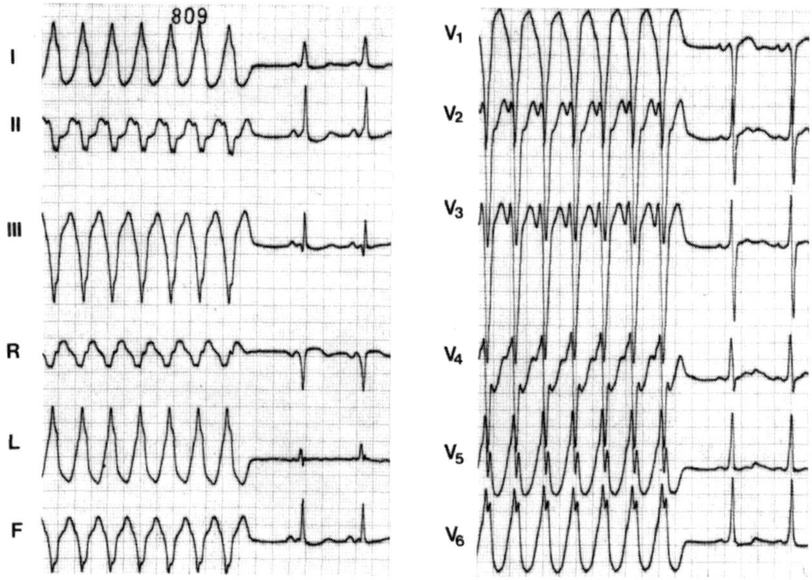

Figure 9.5 An antidromic circus movement tachycardia with AV conduction over a right-sided accessory pathway. The insertion of the accessory pathway in the free wall of the right ventricle results in sequential (first right, then left) ventricular activation and a wide QRS complex.

infarction or myocarditis), ventricular hypertrophy, and muscular disarray (as in hypertrophic cardiomyopathy), also play a role in the QRS width during VT.

It is of interest that a QRS width of more than 0.16 seconds during LBBB-shaped tachycardia argues for a VT [7]. But a QRS width less than such a value may occur in septal VTs. Of course, the QRS width is not helpful in differentiating VT from a tachycardia with AV conduction over a rapidly conducting accessory pathway because such a pathway inserts into the ventricle, leading to eccentric ventricular activation and a wide QRS complex (Fig. 9.5).

The QRS width is also not helpful to distinguish between an SVT with LBBB and an antidromic tachycardia with anterograde conduction over an atriofascicular fiber (Fig. 9.6).

The decrementally conducting pathway can be a short AV structure inserting close to the annulus or a long fiber inserting at or close to the distal RBB. Tachycardias with anterograde conduction over a short decrementally conducting AV pathway usually show a QRS width larger than 0.16 seconds. However, the majority of atriofascicular Mahaim antidromic tachycardias show a QRS complex between 0.12 and 0.14 seconds. Other distinctive findings [20] include an R wave in lead I, rS in V_1, an R/S greater than 1 precordial transition after V_4, and a QRS axis to the left of –30.

An SVT with LBBB can have a QRS width of more than 0.16 seconds under three circumstances: (i) in the presence of preexistent LBBB in the elderly with fibrosis in the bundle-branch system and ventricular myocardium (Fig. 9.7);

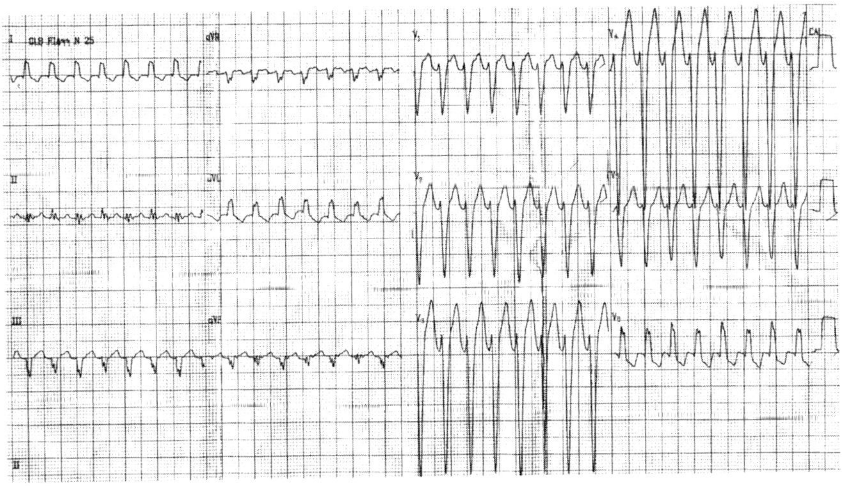

(a)

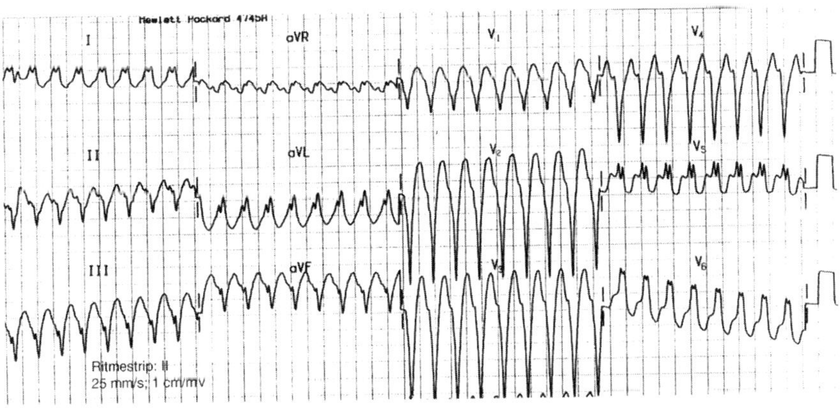

(b)

Figure 9.6 Antidromic tachycardia over a Mahaim fiber. (a) A long atriofascicular pathway inserting in the right bundle is associated with a rather narrow QRS complex (0.12 s). (b) Antidromic tachycardia with anterograde conduction over a short AV pathway with decremental properties inserting close to the annulus is associated with a broader QRS tachycardia (0.16 s).

(ii) when during SVT AV conduction occurs over an accessory AV pathway; and (iii) when class IC drugs (especially flecainide) are present during SVT (Fig. 9.8).

QRS axis in the frontal plane

The QRS axis is not only important to differentiate the broad QRS tachycardia but also to identify its site of origin and etiology. A VT origin in the apicoseptal region of the left ventricle has a superior axis (to the left of –30). An LBBB with

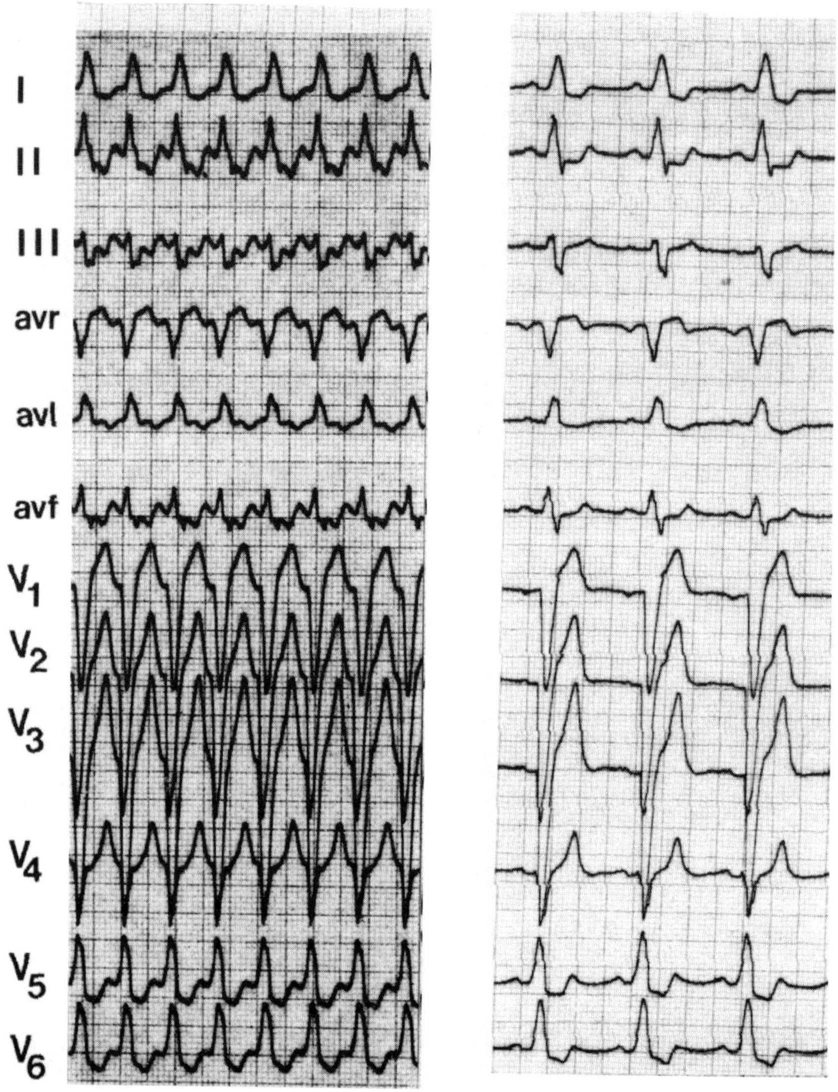

(a) (b)

Figure 9.7 LBBB SVT (a) in a patient with preexistent LBBB (b).

an inferior axis occurs with VT from the right ventricular outflow tract or at the pulmonary artery, just above the pulmonic valve.

Configurational characteristics of the QRS complex

Leads V_1 and V_6

In LBBB-shaped VT, lead V_1 (and/or V_2) (Fig. 9.9) usually shows an initially positive QRS with positivity measuring more than 0.03 seconds; slurring or

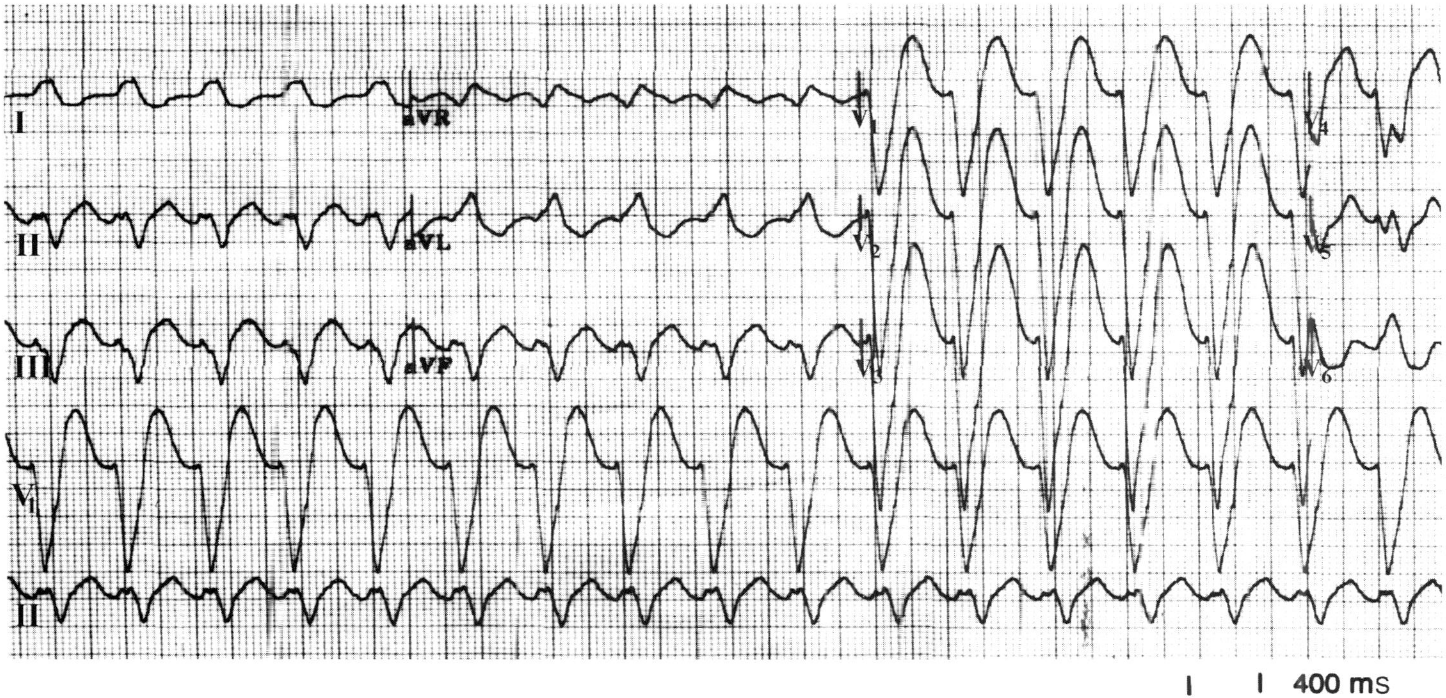

Figure 9.8 Sinus tachycardia presenting as a broad LBBB-shaped QRS tachycardia in a patient using flecainide. Sinus P wave merged with the previous T wave because of a prolonged PR interval.

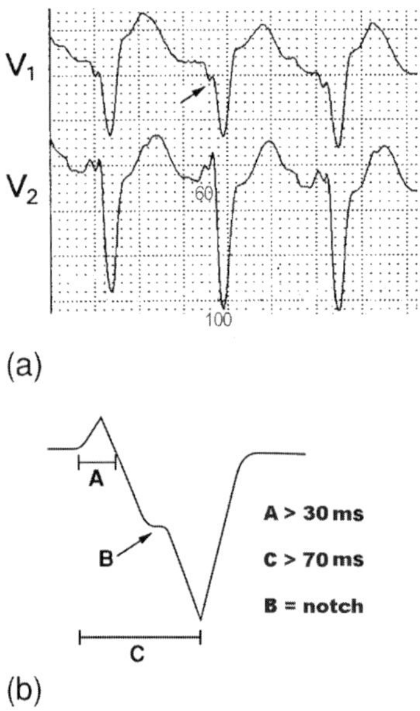

Figure 9.9 (a) V_1 and V_2 from a patient with VT showing an initial R wave width of 60 ms, a notch at the downstroke in V_1, and an interval between the beginning of the QRS to the nadir of the S wave of 100 ms. (b) Findings in lead V_1 and V_2 during LBBB-shaped tachycardia pointing to a ventricular origin.

notching of the downstroke of the S wave; and an interval between the beginning of the QRS axis and the nadir of the S wave of 0.07 seconds or more [10]. When lead V_6 shows a qR pattern during LBBB-shaped tachycardia, VT is very likely. In SVT with LBBB, lead V_1 shows no or minimal initial positivity, a very rapid downstroke of the S wave, and a short interval between the beginning of the QRS and the nadir of the S wave (Fig. 9.10).

LBBB-shaped VTs associated with coronary artery disease are usually adjacent to the interventricular septum and have a higher predictive accuracy for their site of origin than RBBB-shaped VTs. The ECG from an LBBB VT originating in a scar at the apicoseptal region will show a Q wave in leads I and V_6 [21].

Interval onset QRS to nadir of S wave in precordial leads

Brugada *et al.* [12] suggested that an RS interval greater than 100 milliseconds in one or more precordial leads is highly suggestive of VT. One should be careful, however, because such a width may occur in SVT with AV conduction over an accessory pathway, in SVT during administration of drugs that slow intraventricular conduction and in SVT with preexistent BBB, especially LBBB.

Concordant pattern

When all precordial leads show either negative or positive QRS complexes, this is called negative or positive precordial concordance. Negative concordance is diagnostic for VT arising in the apical area of the heart (Fig. 9.11). However,

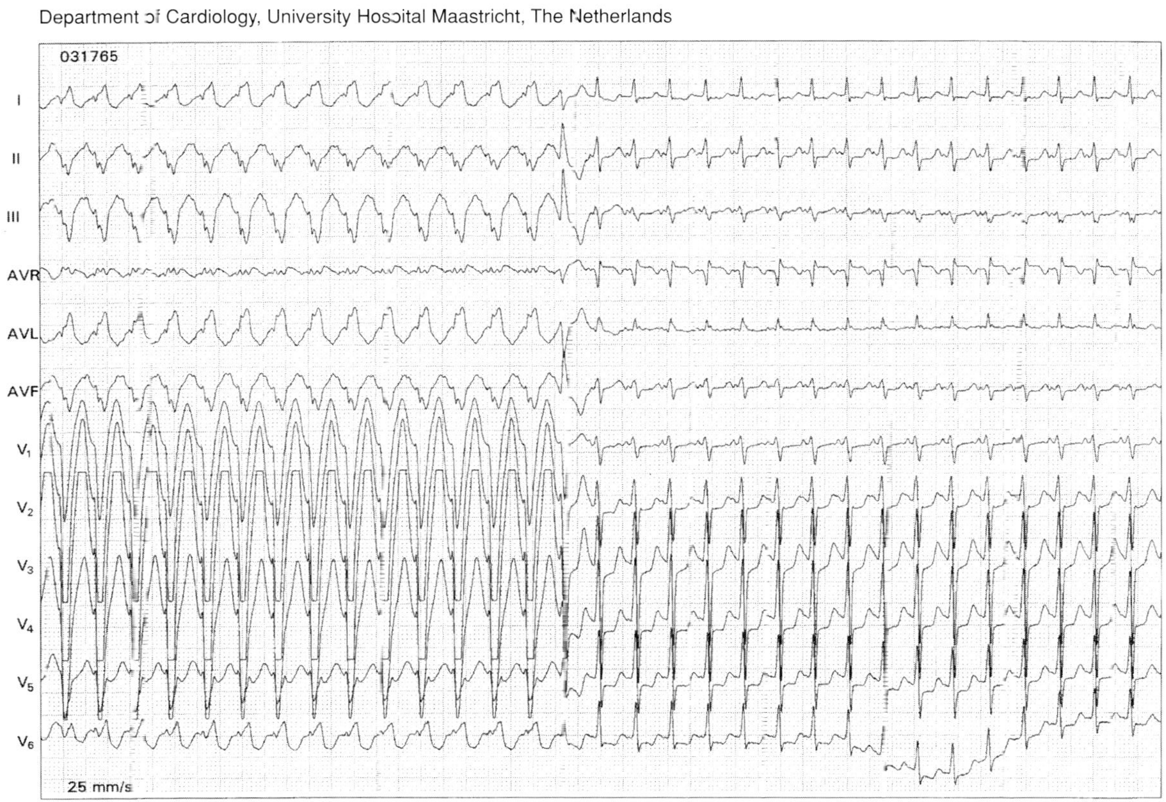

Figure 9.10 SVT with LBBB. The LBBB changes during tachycardia into a narrow QRS following a ventricular premature beat without a change in tachycardia rate. It points to retrograde invasion into the LBB as cause of the LBBB on the left side of the tracing. As described in the text, lead V_1 during LBBB clearly shows signs pointing to a supraventricular origin of the tachycardia.

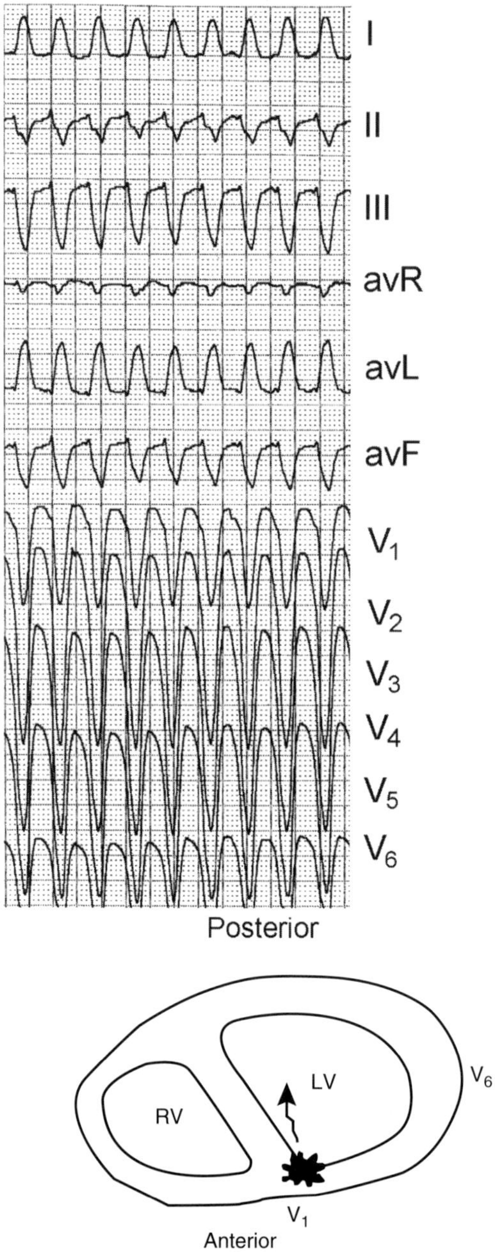

Figure 9.11 Negative concordant precordial pattern. A VT arising in the apical area of the left ventricle results in negative concordance of all precordial leads.

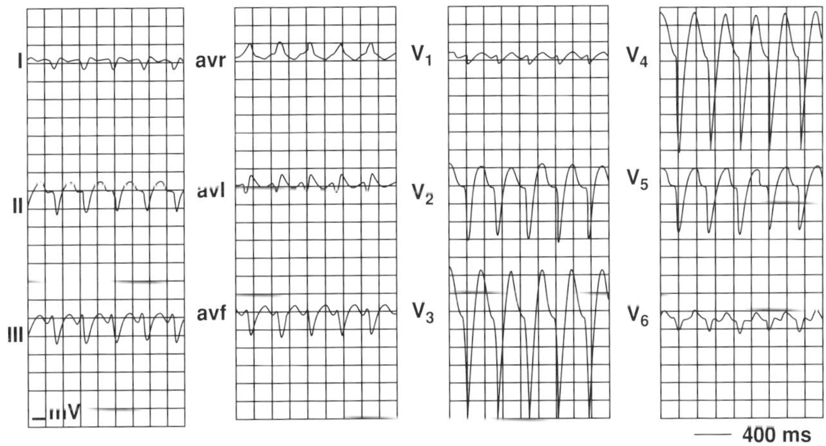

Figure 9.12 Orthodromic AVRT with LBBB showing negative precordial concordance due to abnormal positioning of the heart. Courtesy of Volders *et al.* [22].

an abnormal anatomic position of the heart in a patient with SVT with LBBB can lead to negative concordance in the precordial leads (Fig. 9.12) and a false diagnosis of VT.

One example is *pectus excavatum* where the right ventricle lies completely under the anterolateral precordial area [22]. Positive concordance (all QRS complexes in the precordial leads being positive) can occur in a VT arising in the posterior part of the left ventricle or in a tachycardia with AV conduction over a left posterior accessory pathway.

Tachycardia QRS identical to sinus QRS

When the broad QRS is identical during tachycardia and sinus rhythm, one has to differentiate SVT with preexistent LBBB (Fig. 9.7) from bundle-branch reentrant tachycardia [23]. In diseased hearts, especially when the bundle branches and the interventricular septum are involved, tachycardia may occur based on a circuit with anterograde conduction down one bundle branch and, after septal activation, retrograde conduction over another branch of the bundle-branch system (Fig. 9.13). This type of reentry may occur in patients with anteroseptal myocardial infarction, idiopathic dilated cardiomyopathy, and myotonic dystrophy and in patients after aortic valve surgery and severe frontal chest trauma.

Tachycardia QRS more narrow than sinus QRS

When during tachycardia the QRS is narrower than the one during sinus rhythm, a VT should be diagnosed. This can be explained by the site of origin of the VT close to the interventricular septum, resulting in more simultaneous activation of the ventricles in contrast to the sequential activation of first the right and then the left ventricle in the presence of LBBB during sinus rhythm.

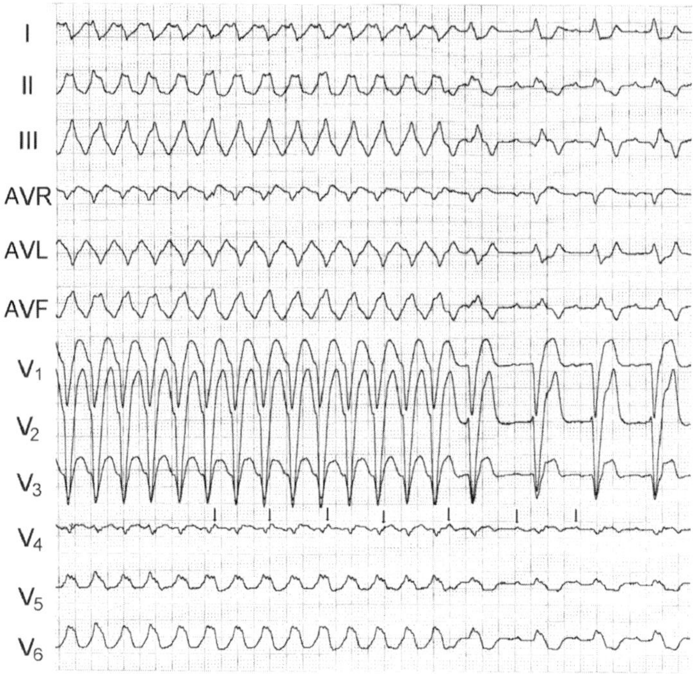

Figure 9.13 Bundle branch reentrant tachycardia. The QRS complexes are identical during tachycardia and sinus rhythm. The PR interval is prolonged during sinus rhythm.

Presence of QR complexes

Coumel *et al.* [24] called attention to the significance of a QR (but not a QS) complex during broad QRS tachycardia, showing that their presence indicates a scar in the myocardium usually caused by myocardial infarction. Figure 9.14 gives an example of QR complexes during an LBBB-shaped VT in a patient with an old inferior myocardial infarction. QR or qR complexes during VT are present in approximately 40% of VTs after myocardial infarction [25].

Etiology of VT

Most VTs have a previous myocardial infarction as their etiology, and, as pointed out, a QR complex during VT can be very helpful to make that diagnosis. However, characteristic ECG patterns can also be found in idiopathic VT [26] and VT in patients with ARVD [27]. Figure 9.15 shows the QRS pattern of idiopathic VT arising close to the outflow tract of the right ventricle.

In some patients, tachycardia does not arise on the endocardial surface of the right ventricular outflow tract but epicardially around the root of the pulmonary valve [28], or in the root of the aorta going to the posterior part of the outflow tract of the right ventricle. An early precordial transition (R/S > 1) or

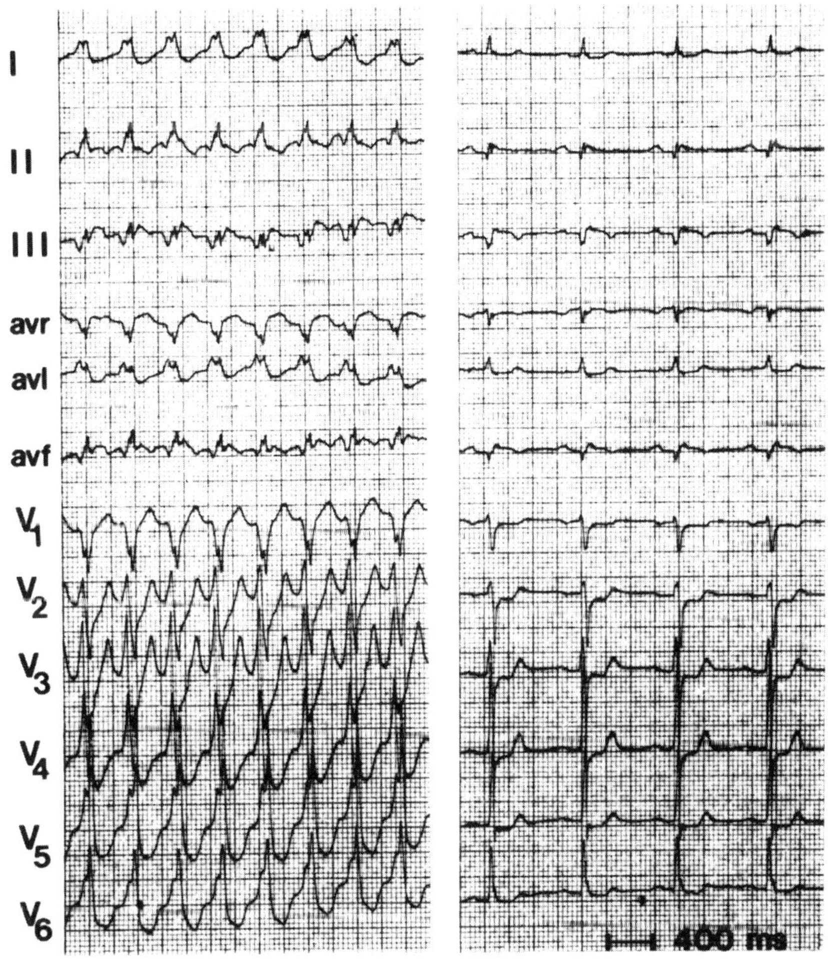

(a) (b)

Figure 9.14 QRS complexes during VT indicating a myocardial scar (QR in leads III and aVF). As shown by the accompanying tracing, during sinus rhythm an inferior wall myocardial infarction is present.

a greater R wave in right precordial leads is consistent with an RV epicardial site of origin [29].

In ARVD, there are three predilection sites in the right ventricle: the inflow tract, the outflow tract, and the apex (Fig. 9.16). While the first two sites have a QRS configuration during tachycardia, which is difficult to differentiate from right ventricular idiopathic VT, left axis deviation in a young person with an LBBB-shaped VT should immediately lead to the suspicion of ARVD (Fig. 9.2a). In fact, an important rule in LBBB-shaped VT with left axis deviation is that cardiac disease should be suspected and that idiopathic right ventricular VT is unlikely.

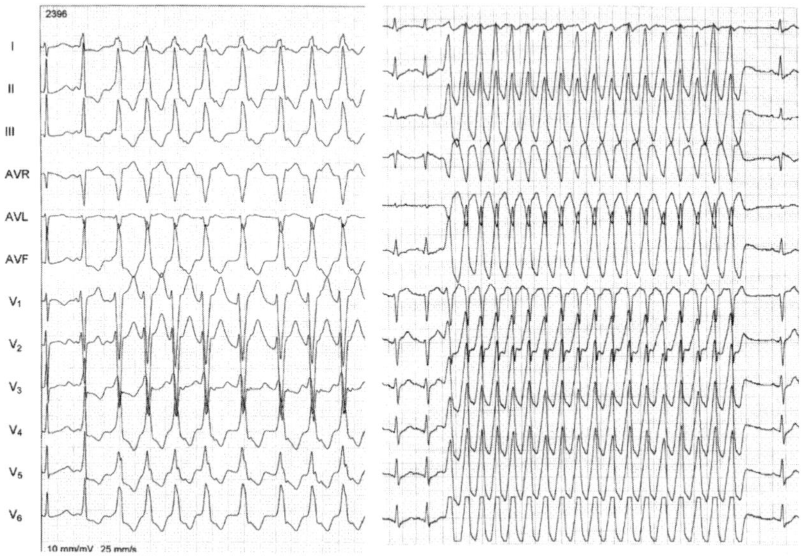

Figure 9.15 Two types of idiopathic VT arising in or close to the outflow tract of the right ventricle. (a) on the lateral part and (b) on the septal side of the right ventricle.

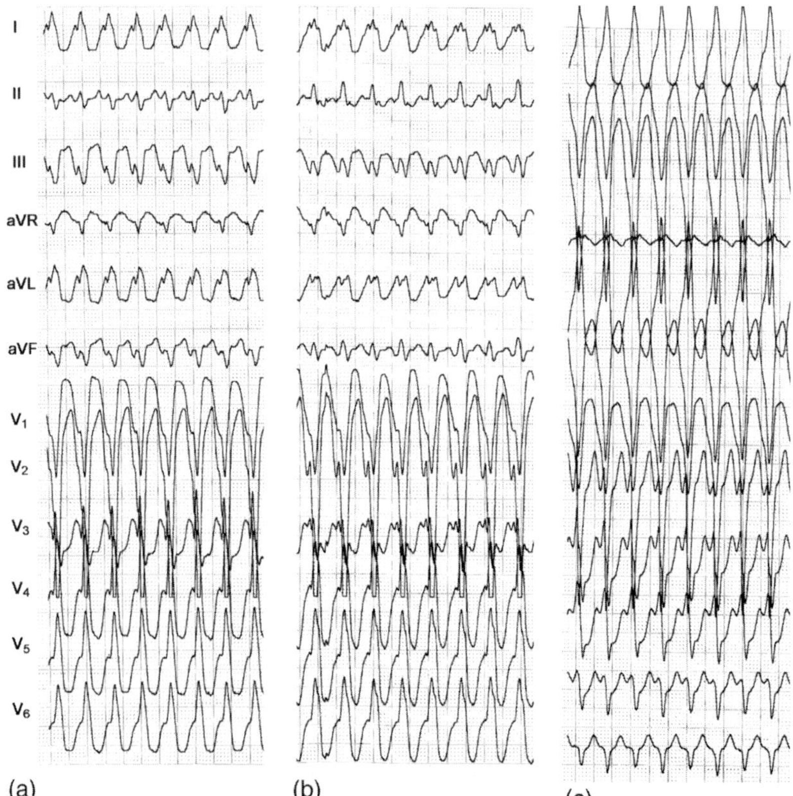

Figure 9.16 Three VTs from a patient with right ventricular dysplasia. VTs (a) and (b) are from the inflow tract, while the VT in (c) originates from the apex of the right ventricle.

Value of the ECG during sinus rhythm

The ECG during sinus rhythm may show changes such as preexistent LBBB, ventricular preexcitation, or an old myocardial infarction, which are very helpful in correctly interpreting the ECG during an LBBB-shaped QRS tachycardia. We have recently described [30] a novel ECG signal suggestive of an atriofascicular fiber in young patients with palpitations, which is an rS pattern in lead III. This pattern can be seen in 2% of normal young persons, but when this rS pattern is associated with the absence of a Q wave in lead I, it is very specific for atriofascicular fibers.

The presence of AV conduction disturbances during sinus rhythm make it very unlikely that a broad QRS tachycardia in that patient has a supraventricular origin and, as discussed, a QRS width during tachycardia narrower than during sinus rhythm points to a VT.

References

1 Bistene A, Sodi-Pallares D, Medrano GA, Pilleggi F. A new approach for the recognition of ventricular premature beats. *Am J Cardiol* 1960;5:358.

2 Kistin AD. Problems in differentiation of ventricular arrhythmias from supraventricular arrhythmia with abnormal QRS. *Prog Cardiovasc Dis* 1966;9:1.

3 Marriott HJL, Sandler JA. Criteria, old and new, for differentiating between ectopic ventricular beats and aberrant ventricular conduction in the presence of atrial fibrillation. *Prog Cardiovasc Dis* 1966;9:18.

4 Massumi RA, Tawakkol AA, Kistin AD. Re-evaluation of electrocardiographic and bedside criteria for diagnosis of ventricular tachycardia. *Circulation* 1967;36:628.

5 Wellens HJJ, Durrer D. Supraventricular tachycardia with left aberrant conduction due to retrograde invasion into the left bundle branch. *Circulation* 1968;38:474.

6 Wellens HJJ. *Electrical Stimulation of the Heart in the Study and Treatment of Tachycardias.* University Park Press, Baltimore; 1971.

7 Wellens HJJ, Bar FWHM, Lie KI. The value of the electrocardiogram in the differential diagnosis of a tachycardia with a widened QRS complex. *Am J Med* 1978;64:27.

8 Wellens HJJ, Brugada P. Diagnosis of ventricular tachycardia from the 12-lead electrocardiogram. *Cardiol Clinics* 1987;5:511.

9 Dongas J, Lehmann MH, Mahmud R, *et al.* Value of pre-existing bundle branch block in the electrocardiographic differentiation of supraventricular from ventricular origin of wide QRS tachycardia. *Am J Cardiol* 1985;55:717.

10 Kindwall KE, Brown J, Josephson ME. Electrocardiographic criteria for ventricular tachycardia in wide complex left bundle branch block morphology tachycardias. *Am J Cardiol* 1988;61:1279.

11 Griffith MJ, de Belder MA, Linker NJ, *et al.* Multivariate analysis to simplify differential diagnosis of broad complex tachycardia. *Brit Heart J* 1991;66:166.

12 Brugada P, Brugada J, Mont L, *et al.* A new approach to the differential diagnosis of a regular tachycardia with a wide QRS complex. *Circulation* 1991;83:1649.

13 Jazayeri MR, Akthar M. Wide QRS complex tachycardia: electrophysiological mechanisms and electrocardiographic features. In: Zipes DP and Jalife J, eds. *Cardiac Electrophysiology: from Cell to Bedside.* Philadelphia: WB Saunders; 1994:990.

14 Nibley C, Wharton JM. Ventricular tachycardias with left bundle branch block morphology. *Pacing Clin Electrophysiol* 1995;18:334.

15 Griffith MJ, Garratt CJ, Mounsey P, Camm AJ. Ventricular tachycardia as default diagnosis in broad complex tachycardia. *Lancet* 1994;343:386.

16 Harvey WP, Ronan JA. Bedside diagnosis of arrhythmias. *Prog Cardiovasc Dis* 1966;8:419.

17 Shimizu A, Ohe T, Takaki H, *et al.* Narrow QRS complex tachycardia with atrioventricular dissociation. *Pacing Clin Electrophysiol* 1988;11:384.

18 Haissaguerre M, Campos J, Marcus FI, *et al.* Involvement of a nodofascicular connection in supraventricular tachycardia with VA dissociation. *J Cardiovasc Electrophysiol* 1994;5:854.

19 Wellens HJJ. Ventricular tachycardia: diagnosis of broad QRS complex tachycardia. *Heart* 2001;86:579.

20 Bardy GH, Fedor JM, German LD, *et al.* Surface electrocardiographic clues suggesting presence of a nodofascicular mahaim fiber. *J Am Coll Cardiol* 1984;3:1161.

21 Miller JM, Marchlinski FE, Buxton AE, Josephson ME. Relationship between the 12-lead electrocardiogram during VT and endocardial site of origin in patients with coronary artery disease. *Circulation* 1988;77:759.

22 Volders PGA, Timmermans C, Rodriguez LM, *et al.* Wide QRS complex tachycardia with negative precordial concordance: always a ventricular origin? *J Cardiovasc Electrophysiol* 2003;14:109.

23 Oreto G, Smeets JL, Rodriguez LM, *et al.* Wide complex tachycardia with atrioventricular dissociation and QRS morphology identical to that of sinus rhythm: a manifestation of bundle branch reentry. *Heart* 1996;76:541.

24 Coumel P, Leclerq JF, Attuel P, Slama R. The QRS morphology in postmyocardial infarction ventricular tachycardia: a study of 100 tracings compared with 70 cases of idiopathic ventricular tachycardia. *Eur Heart J* 1984;5:792.

25 Wellens HJJ. The electrocardiographic diagnosis of arrhythmias. In: Topol E, ed. *Textbook of Cardiovascular Medicine.* Philadelphia: Lippincott, Raven; 1998:1591.

26 Wellens HJJ, Rodriguez LM, Smeets JLRM. Ventricular tachycardia in structurally normal hearts. In: Zipes DP, Jalife J, eds. *Cardiac Electrophysiology- From Cell to Bedside*, 2nd ed. Philadelphia: WB Saunders; 1995:780.

27 Leclerq JF, Coumel PH. Characteristics, prognosis and treatment of the ventricular arrhythmias of right ventricular dysplasia. *Eur Heart J* 1989;10:61.

28 Timmermans C, Rodriguez LM, Crijns HJGM, *et al.* Idiopathic left bundle-branch block-shaped ventricular tachycardia may originate above the pulmonary valve. *Circulation* 2003;108:1960.

29 Ouyang F, Fotuhi P, Ho Sy, *et al.* Repetitive monomorphic ventricular tachycardia originating from the aortic sinus cusp: electrocardiographic characterization for guiding catheter ablation. *J Am Coll Cardiol* 2002;39:500.

30 Sternick EB, Timmermans C, Sosa E, *et al.* The electrocardiogram in sinus rhythm and during tachycardia in patients with anterograde conduction over Mahaim fibers: the role of the "rS" pattern in lead III. *J Am Coll Cardiol* 2004;44:1626.

Index

Note: Page numbers in *italic* refer to figures and/or tables